Reversing Neuropathy

MAKING THE IMPOSSIBLE, POSSIBLE

By Dr. Brian Prax,

DC, CCSP, BCIM, CAFNI

suggestions, procedures, products, and services discussed in this book. Should the reader have any questions concerning the appropriateness of any procedures or products mentioned, the author and publisher strongly suggest consulting with a professional healthcare advisor.

This is the United States of America and we as Americans shall be free to write and say whatever we choose. We respectfully request that you acknowledge that what is written in this book is protected by the First Amendment of the U.S. Constitution. If you cannot agree to the above, then please close this book and do not read any further. Your continued reading is your acknowledgment and agreement to hold harmless everyone from everything.

The information presented herein represents the view of the author as of the date of publication. Because of the rate with which conditions change, the author reserves the right to alter and update his opinion based on the new conditions. This book is for informational purposes only. While every attempt has been made to verify the information provided in this book, neither the author nor his affiliates/partners assume any responsibility for errors, inaccuracies or omissions. Any slights of people or organizations are unintentional.

First Edition

Printed in the U.S.A.
ISBN-13: 978-1974027910
ISBN-10: 1974027910

FOREWORD

We are two decades into the most extraordinary chronic disease epidemic in the history of mankind and the United States is leading an all-out charge to the bottom of the heap on health outcomes. Recently ranked 49th in the world for overall health outcomes, our nation's health is now falling behind war-torn nations like Croatia, and nations in the developing world like Chile. Meanwhile, Americans spend more than double the per capita healthcare cost of any other developed country to achieve these dismal results.

As this book begins, Dr. Brian Prax lays out the extraordinary reality of these epidemics, and accurately identifies many of the convenience lifestyle practices that we have adopted in the last few decades that have engineered the collapse of health in our bodies and that of our nation.

Each of us is now one degree of separation from a family member or close friend that is suffering a premature downward spiral of health. We often watch in amazement, horror, and hopelessness as health seeps out of the body while doctors, with all of our education, diagnostic tools, drug technologies, and treatments, seem unable to bring forth any root cause rationale for the emergence of these disease epidemics, let alone any meaningful solution.

Too many of us are bouncing from specialist to specialist looking for answers to our increasingly desperate frustrations and health challenges, never getting a big picture of how we came to the disorder and dysfunction that we are experiencing in our health or any meaningful solutions for our conditions. Dr. Prax comes to the rescue here to lay out a clear, cause-and-effect picture of how our health has declined. The old adage "knowing the problem is 90% of the battle" is very accurate here. Once we identify the factors that have put us on our path to decline, it is so simple to identify the opposite path toward health and healing.

The choice is then for you to make; are you going to jump the rails on the path of your decline to realize a new potential and quality of life in the days and weeks to come, or are you going to rest in the knowing and make stepwise efforts toward a healthier body in the years to come. Regardless of your trajectory, I am confident you will not be able to stay-the-course on your path of decline once you have gotten through this book.

By picking up this book, you have already identified yourself as someone looking for new answers to long-term problems, and the simplicity of the answers outlined by Dr. Prax makes the opportunity for health too attractive to resist.

As someone likely to be suffering from peripheral neuropathy, you have probably witnessed the 'band-aid' approach to your symptom management – cholesterol drugs, blood pressure drugs, anti-inflammatories, pain medications, anti-depressants, anti-seizure medications, and the list goes on. Each drug class carries its own burden of side effects that reflect the way in which these pharmaceutical agents undermine the biology that we most need to support when wellness begins to decay.

Dr. Prax outlines for us here a stepwise approach to supporting multiple elements of the healing process for the nerves of your body, a plan to reverse your condition at the root of its source. Having practiced integrative medicine alongside Dr. Prax for years, I have witnessed firsthand the power of the multimodality approach that he employs. Like all effective healing, it is most successful and rapid when a problem is addressed from multiple angles. In this way, this book is a one-stop shop for some of the most effective lifestyle practices, technologies, and supplements to support and speed your health recovery.

If your health challenge stopped with you, there would not be the sense of urgency that Dr. Prax and I both feel toward your efforts. The reality is, each subsequent generation since the 1960s is showing an ever-increasing burden of chronic disease, and the occurrence of these conditions happens at a younger age with each of these generations. We are on course to have one in three children with a neurologic deficit by

2035, and the scant 17 years that we have before we hit this crippling state of disease in the children of our nation are going to fly by.

The efforts you make toward reversing your condition and embracing your healing potential is not just a win for your life and welfare, it can be an epicenter of change and education for your entire family and community at large. As such, it is my sincere expectation that the following chapters will empower you to take the necessary steps to change the life you live today, and the future that you can create for yourself and those you love.

Godspeed in health and healing,
Zach Bush, MD
Internal Medicine, Endocrinology and Metabolism, Hospice and Palliative Care

Contents

Chapter 1

My Story

Thank you for picking up this book on how to reverse peripheral neuropathy. I'm Dr. Brian Prax and I've been practicing holistic and functional medicine since 1996, when I earned my Doctor of Chiropractic degree from Life Chiropractic College West in California. My wife, a holistic Pediatric Chiropractor, and I, along with our four children, have lived in Charlottesville, Virginia since 2005.

With my proven neuropathy system, you may be able to reverse your neuropathy. Here's the reality: IT TAKES WORK. Don't let the title of the book fool you. Reversing peripheral neuropathy is not easy, but IT IS POSSIBLE. Don't let your doctors, Big Pharma, therapists, neighbors, family, friends or other naysayers tell you otherwise.

Speaking of naysayers, let me just get something out there right off the bat. Often when I am introduced by my wife or my staff as "Doctor Brian Prax," I'll get the inquiring follow up question; "Oh, you're a doctor; what kind of doctor are you?"

"I'm an 'O' doctor!" I reply.

"An 'O' doctor," what kind of doctor is that?"

I strategically pause and then…. "I'm a……CHI-RO-PRAC-TOR!"

"Ohhhhh!" they exclaim, as if to say, "one of THOOOOOSE kinds of doctors".

All joking aside, there are so many misconceptions about chiropractors I figured I should discuss this right up front. Over the years, we've been labeled as quacks, charlatans, snake oil salesman and more. We seem to be the red-headed stepchildren of Western Medicine. The Cinderellas if you will.

Often, I'll have a patient I'm consulting with say, "Well that sounds good, but I'm gonna check with my "real" doctor. Or, "I'd like to see what my "regular" doctor has to say about that."

I used to be insulted by these comments. You'd think doctors of chiropractic received our doctorates from a Cracker Jack® box! Nowadays, though, I have a different outlook. I suppose that over 20 years of taking this abuse has hardened me, like the forging of metal.

I used to take the time to explain that chiropractors, like medical doctors, have very rigorous education and training. We have clinical rounds, state and national boards to pass too. We have more—way more—training on things natural like nutrition, exercise and, of course chiropractic adjusting than our medical colleagues, whereas they have more training on prescribing medications and surgery.

I used to, that is. Until the truth came out. It first happened in the year 2000. And it happened in one of the most renowned and well-respected journals in the medical profession, none other than the Journal of the American Medical Association. The author, Dr. Barbara Starfield, a medical doctor with a Master's degree in Public Health, unequivocally claimed that medicine is the third leading cause of death in America. Yes, you read that right. <u>MEDICINE IS THE THIRD CAUSE OF DEATH IN AMERICA.</u>

It rocked the world of chiropractic. We were all excited...finally our breakthrough had come. Finally, we'd shine as the natural alternative to the field of medicine. We had been saying for decades, dating back to our founder, D.D. Palmer, in 1895 that medicine is dangerous and a killer. A therapy worthwhile, no doubt, for emergencies and life-threatening cases, but a dangerous one for all things related to healing and wellness.

Our saving grace, though, fell on deaf ears. We wondered why CNN, Fox, NBC, ABC and the other networks didn't jump on such a scandal. What a story, we reasoned. Sensational! Then it dawned on us. Those channels and others are owned by the giant pharmaceutical industry and there's a lot of money to be made on selling their products – medicines.

Think about it. Flip on the TV or radio or just open up the newspaper and take a look at the ads. You'll see the car commercials, sure, but more often than those will be ads for drugs. Sickening too, when you come to realize that the great U.S. of A. is the only country in the entire world (except New Zealand) that directly markets pharmaceutical drugs to consumers. All other countries ban it. You've heard it before..."Ask your doctor if Lyrica is right for you!"

Amazingly, lobbyists have not been able to convince Congress to stop forcing them to state common side effects like "burning, tingling and numbness in the extremities, seizures and death," in their commercials. A commercial I just heard on the internet spent 20 seconds on how great you'd feel taking their drug and the remaining 40 seconds on all of the horrible side effects you should consult your doctor about.

Astoundingly, more research papers from well-known, credible sources continued to pop up. A book, *Death by Medicine,* written by an MD and 3 Ph.D.s came out in 2010 and stated that, when you really look at all the statistics, <u>medicine is the NUMBER ONE CAUSE OF DEATH IN AMERICA.</u>

Yet another research article written by two MDs, Professors of Surgery and Health Policy and

Management at Johns Hopkins Medical School, and published in the respectable BJM (British Medical Journal), stated that medical errors are the third leading cause of death in America. It was published in May 2016. According to the researchers, the coding system used by CDC to record death certificate data doesn't capture things like communication breakdowns, diagnostic errors and poor judgment that cost lives, the study says. To be clear, these "medical errors" do not account for patients that come into the E.R. hanging to life by a thread and then die under a doctor's care. These deaths are doctor mistakes.

Whether medicine is the first or third cause of death doesn't really matter, does it? We can let the researches duke it out on that one, but we can all agree that a healing method should not even be on the list of killers, right? If this is what being a "real" doctor or "regular" doctor means, I want no part of it. In fact, I'm completely okay being your "unreal" doctor or even your "irregular" doctor.

"I've got the Best Doctor in the World"

I can't tell you how many times I have heard a new patient say that they consulted with "the best neurologist" or "the number 1 surgeon in the country." My question to them is always this: "If your doctor is so good, then why are you here consulting with me?" Clearly, even the best medicines and doctors cannot offer ways to reverse certain conditions like peripheral neuropathy.

This is why I have made chronic conditions like peripheral neuropathy my top priority to master and learned everything I can, beyond medicine, to improve and even reverse. I know, even after reading this book, there will still be naysayers that'll hold onto the old dogma of "it can't be done" or "nothing can help neuropathy" or "you're just going to have to learn to live with it." You just have to think outside of the box. I love Albert Einstein's famous quote, "No problem can be solved from the same level of consciousness that created it." So, you may have to incorporate Apple's famous tagline; "Think Different."

If you have already exhausted your willingness to try what traditional medicine has to offer for your condition, you've picked up the right book. In the pages that follow, you will learn how you got where you are and how to reverse that. I've found that typically the neuropathy puzzle consists of many pieces. Some will get lucky and find the one piece, like B vitamins often peddled on the internet. Others may bump across a diet that could literally solve the problem, but for most, I have found that we must get ALL of the neuropathy pieces together to completely heal this debilitating condition.

One thing that I can promise you though is this: you will NEVER be able to medicate yourself out of neuropathy. Medicines like Gabapentin (common trade name is Neurontin), Lyrica (Pregabalin) or Amitriptyline (Elavil) only mask the pain at best. At worst, they do not help with the pain and create side effects that are so bad, the user ends up in a worse condition.

By the way, did you know that Americans consume over 75% of all the medications in the world?! That's a big eye opener, especially when you consider that we only comprise 5% of the world's population! What about this statistic? Americans pay way more for so-called "health care" than just about any other nation in the world ($9403 in 2014 and rising), yet we are ranked 50th out of 55 nations by a recent Bloomberg Healthcare Efficiency Index.[1] If our medical system REALLY WORKED to fix conditions like peripheral neuropathy, we would be the healthiest nation in the world, not the 50th.

So, if you are looking for something different, if you really are sick and tired of Western Medicine's Drug and Cut paradigm, then you have come to the right place. My neuropathy reversal program has an 85% success rate. Bet you are wondering how that's possible? Let me explain...

First, I need to define "success." For me, that means anywhere from 60% to 100% better based on the

---

[1]https://www.bloomberg.com/news/articles/2016-09-29/u-s-health-care-system-ranks-as-one-of-the-least-efficient

patient's assessment. For others, you may need to set realistic expectations. If your condition is so far advanced that you can barely feel your feet or hands, maybe "success" would mean being able to sleep through the night without being woken up by tingling or pain.

For others, it could mean that the burning pain in your feet is 25% better. Second, you must know that not every case of neuropathy will respond to the natural therapies we'll discuss in this book. Some people will not get better because their condition is so far deteriorated, it's irreversible. Sometimes a case is just too advanced – there's too much damage to expect even the slightest amount of recovery.

Some cases will need other therapies – yes, maybe even drugs or surgery. Some of you may have conditions like Multiple Sclerosis, GuillainBarré syndrome, Polio, or other conditions (that have yet to be discovered) complicating or causing your neuropathy. Can those be fixed? It just depends on how progressed your condition is, but don't ever give up. Throwing in the towel will never change a single thing. We know that for sure. Even if you followed the neuropathy protocols discussed in this book and, worst case scenario, it doesn't get better, your entire body will be healthier and without any negative side effects. It's a win-win situation.

I hope this has given you an idea of who I am and how passionate I am about helping you reverse this debilitating condition. I am straight to the point, honest, realistic, and transparent. Do you want to see if this program can help you? Then keep reading! Keep an open mind, take good notes, and follow the recommendations.

Chapter 2

Who's to Blame for America's Health Crisis?

Case Study

Mary S (77 years) came to my office complaining of carpal tunnel syndrome (numbness and weakness in her hands), lower back pain, sciatica, hip pain, and severe insomnia. "My fingers were numb, and my legs had sciatica – they were keeping me up all night. It was just pain and aching. I went on the program [which includes a] really healthy diet. It's more like a lifestyle. It's watching what I put in my mouth – I'm eating real human food. I have lost 7lbs in about 4 weeks. I am more alert. I'm not having my gastrointestinal problems. At 6 weeks into the 12-week program, I am feeling 50% better. I'm real pleased with my progress. I needed help! [I learned that] we can regenerate nerve activity. Most people don't know that. Their physicians don't tell them what's possible because they don't even know."

By the end of her program she was calling the office to excitedly tell my staff and I that she had not just one, but 2 nights of painless sleep for the first time in a very long time. Her doctor reduced her medications, her balance greatly improved, and the lower lumbar pain was "75% better". I think she best summed it up with this statement. "Super, super, super! The best! 10 stars!"

People tend to think of today's health crisis in the United States as a health *insurance* crisis. Fingers are pointed at many parties for the current state of affairs:

- The government, for the lack of universal and affordable health insurance.
- Pharmaceutical companies, for the ever-increasing price of prescription drugs.
- Health care industry, for poorly managed health care practices.
- The food industry, because lower-income individuals are practically forced to purchase cheap, highly processed, unhealthy foods.

Although each of these parties has a hand in perpetuating the crisis, none of them is the actual cause. The real reason behind the health care crisis is each individual's poor choices and lifestyle, mostly in the areas of food, exercise, and stress management. This leads to health-related issues like cancer, heart disease, metabolic syndrome, stroke, diabetes, and so much more.

Whether we like it or not, each one of us must take personal responsibility for our health. This means educating ourselves about the choices that will make a positive change for us and for those we love.

Biggest Health Issue Is Big Indeed

Perhaps the most significant health issue in the United States is obesity. In fact, it is at epidemic proportions. Consider these statistics:

- Among Americans age 20 and older, 154.7 million are overweight or obese.[2]
- Recently, the number of obese people has outnumbered those who are overweight.
- More than two-thirds (68.8 percent) of adults are overweight or obese.
- More than one-third (35.7 percent) of adults are considered to be obese.[3]
- 18% of deaths in America are associated with obesity. These deaths stem primarily from type

---

[2] Go AS, Mozaffarian D, Roger VL, Benjamin EJ, Berry JD, Borden WB, Bravata DM, Dai S, Ford ES, Fox CS, Franco S, Fullerton HJ, Gillespie C, Hailpern SM, Heit JA, Howard VJ, Huffman MD, Kissela BM, Kittner SJ, Lackland DT, Lichtman JH, Lisabeth LD, Magid D, Marcus GM, Marelli A, Matchar DB, McGuire DK, Mohler ER, Moy CS, Mussolino ME, Nichol G, Paynter NP, Schreiner PJ, Sorlie PD, Stein J, Turan TN, Virani SS, Wong ND, Woo D, Turner MB; on behalf of the American Heart Association Statistics Committee and Stroke Statistics Subcommittee. Heart disease and stroke statistics—2013 update: a report from the American Heart Association. Circulation. 2013;127:e6-e245.

[3] https://www.niddk.nih.gov/health-information/health-statistics/overweight-obesity

2 diabetes, hypertension, heart disease, liver disease, cancer, dementia, and depression.[4]

How Did the Obesity Problem Get So Big?

Early in the 20th century, the American diet was entirely different from what it is today. If you could hop in a time machine and peek onto the shelves at the local store your grandparents shopped at, you would see produce, living plants, seeds, and grains. A quick walk to the local butcher and you'd find all natural, fresh, organic, grass-raised, grass-finished beef, chicken, turkey and more...oh, and it would all be local. Nowadays, you have to be a food scientist to know what the "right" foods are to buy.

Here's what you'll find in modern grocery stores:
- hormone injected meats
- highly refined, starchy foods
- processed foods
- fast foods
- junk foods
- sugar, sugar and more sugar

With these "modern" food choices comes a completely different diet – "The Standard American Diet," aka S.A.D. The foods found in the S.A.D. diet are entirely out of balance.

---

[4] Masters, Ryan, PhD. News. Columbia University Mailman School of Public Health. "Obesity Kills More Americans Than Previously Thought". N.p., 15 Aug. 2013.

Incredibly, billions of dollars have been spent on various studies in a quest to find the causes and solutions for obesity. But the real answer is sitting in plain sight in homes across America: specifically, in the kitchens and on the couches.

The answer to the obesity crisis and the health care crisis in general is simple – return to a more natural diet rich in fresh fruits and vegetables, unprocessed meats, nuts, seeds, good fats and fiber while avoiding processed foods (and being active every day). You know what I call this? **A normal human diet.** Here's a great rule of thumb – if God, or nature, made the food, it's probably going to be good for you. If man or the food industry tinkered with nature's food or made their own food-like product, IT'S BAD FOR YOU!

Trying to Make the Perfect Food Better

Food companies work tirelessly at making nature's already perfect foods better by refining them and processing them and adding chemicals to them. These food products are loaded with extra salt, sugar, artificial flavors, preservatives, and other chemicals. They are also missing vital nutrients and vitamins that are stripped away during processing. This adding and subtracting from our food is a recipe for disaster and obesity. All of this tinkering has created an American diet that is high in calories and, at the same time, deficient in nutrients – this is the perfect recipe for obesity. It's really quite the paradox how most of us are eating way too many calories and, at the same time, are starving and undernourished. When our bodies are not getting enough of the vitamins, minerals and other necessary, life-supporting nutrients we need to thrive, we keep getting signals from the brain to eat more! So, we eat more of those empty calories and keep getting fatter and fatter and sicker and sicker.

Cutting corners

So why does the food industry go through all the trouble and expense of adding all of this unnatural stuff to our food...wouldn't that be *more* expensive? In a word, the answer is...money. Yes, it's *all about the money*.

Let's take meat for example. You see, the land that the cattle, chickens, pigs, and other animals graze on is expensive and to do it right, each animal needs a certain amount of land, and it's a lot more than you'd think. Put too many cows in one pasture, and they'll nibble that grass right down to the dirt, leaving it barren. Rain and wind will erode the land making it not suitable for growing grass. No grass means no animals – get it? So, what should the rancher do? You gotta make money, right? I mean, you're in business after all.

Well, who needs all that expensive land, the tending and constant repairing of the fences, rounding up your herd and all? Why don't we just build big barns and feed all of the cows in one spot? Way more efficient, yes?

There's a problem though. That many cows under one roof is a breeding ground for disease. But not when you can just put antibiotics in their food. And, while we're at it, let's just put in some growth hormones and steroids to make them grow faster. You see, ranchers are paid by the pound, not for the *quality* of the meat. So, the faster you can get them to market, the more money you can make.

It's pretty much the same for all other animals too. Pigs, sheep, chickens, turkeys and even fish (did you know that nowadays about half of the world's seafood comes from fish farms – which means they are held in large cages, fed grain, legumes, antibiotics and even pesticides). What do you think happens to an animal when it is not fed its normal diet? Well, it's the same for cows and fish as it is for humans. We all get sick! We can all *survive* on these substances, but we cannot *thrive*.

Sugar Blues

Sugar Blues is a book by William Dufty that was released in 1975. A bestseller, Dufty goes into detail about the history of sugar. Consider this from his book.

The status of sugar, as a product of refining, was compared to drugs:

> Heroin is nothing but a chemical. They take the juice of the poppy and they refine it into opium and then they refine it to morphine and finally to heroin....

> Sugar is nothing but a chemical. They take the juice of the cane or the beet and then refine it to molasses and then they refine it to brown sugar and finally to strange white crystals.[5]

The average American consumes 150 POUNDS of sugar every year – compared to just two pounds consumed on average in the year 1700. That's 75 times as much![6] We are just not engineered to eat this much sugar.

Hidden Sugar

I often tell my patients that we must look for *all* forms of sugar, the obvious and the hidden forms. I say, "It's not what's on your plate that's the main issue, but what your body *does with what's on your plate*." Take bread for example – even the whole grain bread that we are told is so healthy for us. As another refined food, grains, like wheat will often turn into sugar in the blood faster than table sugar itself.

Glycemic Index

The "Glycemic Index" (GI) represents the rise in a person's blood sugar level two hours after consumption of the food. Basically, it measures how fast a food is converted into blood sugar, also known as glucose. Glucose on the GI is rated at 100, so let's compare:

---

[5]https://en.wikipedia.org/wiki/Sugar_Blues page 22
[6]https://www.dhhs.nh.gov/dphs/nhp/documents/sugar.pdf

Table sugar has a GI of 65 and is considered to be "medium" on the list (56-69) and we just discussed how bad sugar is for you, but ponder these other commonly eaten foods (and in many cases "staples" of the S.A.D.)
Table

• Sugar 65	• Macaroni and Cheese (Kraft®) 64
• Corn flakes 81	
• Grape Nuts® 75	• Soda crackers 74
• Instant oatmeal, average 79	• Graham Crackers 74
	• White rice, boiled 72
• Average bagel 72	• Couscous 65
• Aunt Jemima Waffles® 76	• M&M's®, peanut 33
	• Fruit Roll-Ups® 99
• Average hamburger bun 61	• Cranberry juice cocktail 68
• White bread 75	• Coca-Cola 63
• Whole wheat bread 69	• Gatorade, orange flavor 89
• Baked russet potato 111	

Now, take another look at those numbers and compare them with the GI of sugar. Many of the very foods that we are told are so "heart healthy" or "digestive healthy" (whole wheat bread, oatmeal, rice) actually turn into blood sugar faster than table sugar itself. "How could that be?" You ask? Great question. Here's a little chemistry. All food must be broken down into their simplest molecules for the body to do things with. They are broken down into amino acids, fatty acids or glucose. So, here's the take-home message. It's not what's on our plate that is important but what your body does with what's on your plate.

Luckily, our body has a mechanism to deal with all this sugar and it's called insulin. It's a hormone that is produced by the pancreas. When the brain detects high levels of blood glucose (because you just ate a couple pieces of whole wheat toast), it signals the pancreas to release insulin. Insulin basically removes the glucose from the blood bringing it back to an optimal level.

Since glucose is a form of energy, the body does not want to get rid of it, so it stores it for later usage…Here's the kicker. Where do you think the body stores it? If you said, "fat," then you were right. It literally converts the blood sugar into fat and packs them throughout your body. So, when there's a famine, or you skip a meal or two, it has energy ready to use.

Therein lies our obesity problem in America. We eat WAY too much sugar and way too many foods that convert into sugar. Flour and cereal products provided more calories per day for the average American than any other food group in 2010. Fruit and vegetable and dairy products provided smaller shares of calories per day for the average American. A healthy body needs a diet high in vitamins, minerals, enzymes, and antioxidants. It's the best way to make sure your body can correctly digest food, absorb nutrients, regulate cell function, and keep your body fueled up.

When your body doesn't have the nutrients it needs, the aging process speeds up. Aging doesn't just mean gray hair and wrinkles – we are talking about all the diseases associated with aging, such as:

- Coronary Heart Disease (CHD): About 610,000 people die of heart disease in the United States each year–that's 1 in every 4 deaths.[7]

- Heart disease costs the United States about $207 billion each year. This total includes the cost of health care services, medications, and lost productivity.[8]

- Stroke: In 2016, strokes caused one of each 20 deaths in the United States. On average, every 40 seconds, someone in the United States has a stroke. Every four minutes, someone dies from a stroke.[9]

---

[7]Mozzafarian D, Benjamin EJ, Go AS, et al. on behalf of the American Heart Association Statistics Committee and Stroke Statistics Subcommittee. Heart disease and stroke statistics—2016 update: a report from the American Heart Association. *Circulation*. 2016;133:e38-e360.

[8]Mozzafarian D, Benjamin EJ, Go AS, et al. on behalf of the American Heart Association Statistics Committee and Stroke Statistics Subcommittee. Heart disease and stroke statistics—2016 update: a report from the American Heart Association. *Circulation*. 2016;133:e38-e360.

[9]"Stroke Statistics." Centers for Disease Control and Prevention. <https://www.cdc.gov/stroke/facts.htm>

- High Blood Pressure: About 75 million American adults (29%) have high blood pressure—that's one of every three adults.[10]

- Cancer: In 2012, there were approximately 13.7 million Americans with a history of cancer. Some of these men and women were cancer-free and others still had evidence of cancer and could be undergoing treatment. In 2013, there were expected to be 1,660,290 new cancer cases.[11]

- Osteoporosis: more than 53 million people either already have osteoporosis or are at high risk due to low bone mass, placing them at risk for more serious bone loss and fractures.[12]

- Diabetes: Data from the 2014 CDC Fact Sheet states that 29 million people in the United States (9.3 percent) have diabetes. Another 86 million adults – more than one in three U.S. adults – have prediabetes[13]). The total cost of diagnosed diabetes in the United States in 2012 was $245 billion.[14]

---

[10] "High Blood Pressure Facts." Centers for Disease Control and Prevention.
<https://www.cdc.gov/bloodpressure/facts.htm>
[11]American Cancer Society. Cancer Facts & Figures 2013. Atlanta: American Cancer Society; 2013.
[12]"Osteoporosis." NIHSeniorHealth.
[13]https://www.cdc.gov/features/diabetesfactsheet
[14]"Diabetes Statistics." Diabetes Basics. American Diabetes Association, 2013.

- Peripheral Neuropathy: Improper diet is a large component of all types of neuropathy.

In 2016, the United States was reported to spend over ten thousand dollars per person on health care.[15] It is hard to believe that there are people dying of an inadequate diet in the United States when there is a surplus of food, but it's true and, according to the "experts," there appears to be little hope of reversing the trend.

Considering that we are ranked 50th of 55 nations in the health care arena, something is wrong. I contend that it is our approach to health that's the problem. What if we actually supported healthy lifestyles instead of simply treating the symptoms associated with a loss of health?[16]

People like to think that modern medicine is the answer to the health care crisis. But experts in the field of medicine realize that despite the use of advanced technology, there has been no decline in the health crisis. The real answer does not rely on the *treating of symptoms*, but in the *prevention* of disease and promotion of health.

---

[15]Ricardo Alonso-Zaldivar, Associated Press *July 13, 2016*.
[16](https://www.bloomberg.com/news/articles/2016-09-29/u-s-health-care-system-ranks-as-one-of-the-least-efficient)

One of the best ways to prevent disease is living a healthy lifestyle. For many people, understanding what constitutes a healthy lifestyle is daunting. Other people know exactly what "healthy living" means, but they are not willing to commit to making the necessary lifestyle changes. Committing to choices like these simply sounds like too much of a hassle:

1. Eat well – Kick the S.A.D. diet out of your life and replace it with a diet filled with fresh fruits and vegetables, lean meats and fish, healthy fats, nuts and seeds.
2. Exercise well – Exercising just 30 minutes three times per week will promote heart health, help you lose weight by increasing your metabolism, build strong bones, boost your immune system and stimulate your nervous system.
3. Sleep well – Most cell repairs and memory assimilation happen during sleep. Most people need seven to eight hours of sleep each night in order to function at their best.
4. Live well – Believe it or not, kindness and love, as well as having a set of principles to guide your life, will help you to be healthier and live longer.
5. Optimal Nervous System Health – Everything that goes on in our body begins with the nervous system. Ridding your body of blockages in the nervous system can help you reach your full potential.

The Good News and the Bad News

Let me be blunt. For most neuropathies, YOU are to blame. YOU got YOU to where you are at this very moment based on what YOU have done to yourself over the course of your lifetime. YOU decided what to feed yourself. YOU decided how to respond to illnesses or injuries. YOU decided to exercise regularly or not at all. The burden of achieving good health falls squarely on your own shoulders. That's the bad news…but also, it's the good news. Since you are where you are based on what you've done, then you can make new choices, RIGHT NOW, and get different results. The good news is that your body is a marvelous being that CAN heal. If you do not like where you are and can swallow the PILL that you created it, you can change what the direction you are heading!

You cannot rely on others to watch out for your health. I'm sure your doctor is a great guy or gal, but s/he can never care more about you than you can. You need to be the strongest advocate for yourself. You cannot find good health at the doctor's office or in the pharmacy. You will NEVER be able to medicate your way out of peripheral neuropathy – we know that for a fact. Drugs, for the most part, only cover up your symptoms. You won't find good health in the unnatural food aisles of the grocery store or in fast food restaurants. Good health can only be found when you commit to a healthy lifestyle.

By taking care of your body now, learning everything you can to make good choices, and finding practitioners who promote the prevention of disease and promotion of health you will be well on your way to a healthier you.

A Big Pill to Swallow

If you can swallow this pill I'm about to give you, you'll be on your way to curing your neuropathy. Here goes: For most kinds of neuropathy, YOU are the underlying cause. Well, you and your doctor. You see, for the vast majority of these cases, it is your lifestyle that killed your nerves. I blame your doctor, but I guess I really shouldn't, because, for most of them, they have no clue how to foster a healthy human being. They are excellent at diagnosing disease and prescribing medicines to help you to feel better and that is the practitioner you go to in a life-threatening condition like stroke, heart attack or trauma. But when it comes to healing – no way! You can't heal yourself by medicating yourself and, as I've said before, you will not be able to drug yourself out of peripheral neuropathy. Darn, because I know how easy it is to take a pill but what it really takes to heal damaged nerves is not that easy.

Who else is to blame?

Alright, it's not ALL your fault. After all, none of our parents were handed The Human Manual like you got with your car, right? Your parents, and eventually you, had to figure it out. You did so with information that society gave you –information from your doctor, family, friends, and the media. If what you were told- day in and day out from the time you were born was to drug your symptoms, that what you eat doesn't really matter and exercise is for the birds, well, that's the advice that you'd most likely follow.

Brainwashed Americans

I often joke with my workshop attendees that the average American household has 2.93 TVs, 2.28 cars, and two washing machines. They get the TVs and cars, but two washing machines? Yes, I say. One of those is your regular washing machine for clothes, and the other is the brainwashing machine called your TV. Did you know that there are only two countries in the world, the United States and New Zealand, which allow pharmaceutical companies to directly market to consumers? The rest of the world governments have evidently determined that this type of marketing is unethical, immoral and even dangerous.

Look, the pharmaceutical industry is just that...an industry. Their top priority is to make money. Think I'm joking? Consider this. "Ad spending for the U.S. healthcare industry in 2015 hit a record \$9 billion, up a record 11%."[17] How could they spend so much money? It takes money to make money, they say. This industry has a 21% profit margin which is huge, making it by far the most profitable industry of all.

---

[17]http://gaia.adage.com/images/bin/pdf/KantarHCwhitepaper _complete.pdf

TV marketing is by far the most effective usage of the industry's dollars, but the internet (websites, blogs, social media, etc) is showing a great return on their investment as well. And, let's not forget about all the other mediums of advertising like newspaper, magazines, radio and more. Have they brainwashed us with their constant bombardment of advertising? To quote the infamous Adolf Hitler; "If you tell a big enough lie, and tell it frequently enough, it will be believed."

So, let's take a moment for introspection. Take a look in your medicine cabinet or on your counter. How many medications are you taking? Do you know what all of them are for? Have you looked up or had a serious discussion with your doctor about their potential side effects? Did you realize that many of them have side effects of peripheral neuropathy, like burning, tingling and numbness in the extremities? How about dizziness, vertigo and balance issues. Did you realize that the very medications that you are being prescribed could be leading contributors to your neuropathy? Remember the stats from the introduction of this book that Americans comprise 5% of the world's population and we consume over 75% of all medications in the world? And that we only rank 50th in terms of "healthy nations"? What about the stat that says that we spend more on so called health care than any other nation in the world? Are you starting to wonder how you got into such a predicament?

But, on a positive note, let's listen to the sage advice of the famous musician, Willie Nelson, "Once you replace negative thoughts with positive ones, you'll start having positive results."

Chapter 3

The Crisis Care Dilemma

Case Study

Jessica is my back-office assistant, and when she began working for me, she was 34 and looked to be the picture of health. After taking a closer look at her new patient assessment forms and her history during her initial exam, it was discovered that she had a 15-year history of kidney disease and an autoimmune disease that has yet to be named by Western Medicine.

She explained that any time she became ill – like the common cold – hives would break out across her chest and, depending on the severity of the illness, they would spread across her whole body, swelling her eyes and face and on numerous occasions, closing off her airway. Essentially, a bad cold carried the potential of deadly consequences.

She had also undergone a full double mastectomy at age 32 for breast disease. When asked about her eating habits, it became pretty clear that dietary changes needed to be made. She was a self-proclaimed chocoholic and junkaholic. Sweets, processed foods, wheat, dairy…it was all there and in excess. She knew her diet was poor but because she could "get away" with eating what she wanted without it showing up on her waistline.

After years of tests, emergency visits, five surgeries, loads of antibiotic treatments for infections and autoimmune flare-ups, and a continual desperate search for answers, not one of the many "REAL DOCTORS" and specialists she saw ever asked her about her diet. Not even one of them.

After 30 days of my anti-inflammatory diet (to be covered in chapter 6), her symptoms began to dissolve and we discovered that her immune reactions were to rice and cheese (a staple of her diet). After one year of a clean diet (and without rice and cheese) she happened to come down with a bad cold... "Uh oh" was her immediate statement. And, do you know what? For the first time in over a decade, she did not have an autoimmune reaction – no rash, no EpiPen, no emergency room. Standard American Diet: 0. Optimal Human Diet: 1.

The Top 3 Causes of Death in the U.S.

#1. Cardiovascular Disease (Deaths: 596,577)
#2. Cancer (Deaths: 576,691)
#3. **Medicine** (Deaths: 440,000)

Modern medicine is crisis-focused and by most accounts, it's the best in the world at that. It runs on the philosophy that aging is the decline phase of life. We are born, we live, we get sick, and we die. But it doesn't have to be that way! That's the first mindset switch we need to make. Instead of thinking of our bodies as vessels destined and designed for deterioration and disease, think of it as being meant for continuous progress. Yes, we all age, and we will all eventually die. But how would the rest of your life be different if you decided to live up to your physical potential?

Think about it.

Are you motivated to be well right now, or will you be far more motivated to be well when you get sick and your comfortable living is taken away from you? Sadly, we only tend to find our motivation when something goes wrong. It's far easier to choose cheeseburgers and couch time over healthier choices –until all those bad choices finally create a disaster for our health.

Convenience is the American Way

Really it all comes down to convenience. Most Americans are trained to be lazy – and businesses cater to our desires. We want our food, coffee, pills and even our health fast, convenient and cheap. Drive-throughs, fast food, fast coffee and Amazon. All fast and all as cheap as possible. And speaking of getting healthy, it is way easier to just pop a pill rather than eating great food day in, day out and actually exercising. Jeez, it takes so much time to make good food and go to the gym, you know?

That's the real cause of the vast majority of diseases we are dealing with today: lifestyle choices. We *should* be motivated every day to live a lifestyle that allows us to thrive, maintain, and enjoy a fantastic quality of life and that's what the wellness movement is all about: seeking wellness instead of seeking cures, each and every day. There is no medication, special lotion, potion, surgery, or injection that will regain our health. I've always said to my patients; "You can't medicate yourself into perfect health. It takes hard work and the right decisions – everyday."

What Is Wellness Care?

More and more people are coming to realize that focusing on their wellness could allow them to live healthier, longer lives. They are demanding that their health care providers work with them on wellness plans that prevent disease rather than just treating symptoms. There is evidence of this shift all around us:

- Organic and local foods are becoming the preferred produce option in America and around the world. The USDA's National Farmers Market Directory's listings have increased by more than 61% from 2008 to

2013.[18] And the number of Farmer's markets continues to grow each year.

- The Veterans Administration has committed to implementing alternative therapies to help veterans deal with pain and avoid possible opioid painkiller addictions.[19]

- According to the National Center for Complementary and Integrative Health, in 2007, approximately 38% of American adults used some form of complementary or alternative medicine treatment.[20]

- The majority of U.S. adults—68 percent—take dietary supplements.[21]

- Part of the wellness revolution has been a shift in the relationship between primary care

---

[18] "News Release." *USDA Celebrates National Farmers Market Week, August 4-10.* United States Department of Agriculture, 5 Aug. 2013. Web. 02 Aug. 2015.
http://www.usda.gov/wps/portal/usda/usdahome?contentid=2013%2F08%2F0155.xml
[19] "Office of Public and Intergovernmental Affairs." News Releases -. VA Office of Public and Intergovernmental Affairs, 25 Feb. 2014. Web. 02 Aug. 2015.
<http://www.va.gov/opa/pressrel/pressrelease.cfm?id=2529>
.
[20]"The Use of Complementary and Alternative Medicine in the United States."
<https://nccih.nih.gov/research/statistics/2007/camsurvey_fs1.htm>
[21]"Most U.S. Adults Take Dietary Supplements, According to New Survey." 2015 CRN CONSUMER SURVEY ON DIETARY SUPPLEMENTS.
http://www.crnusa.org/CRNconsumersurvey/2015/.

doctors and patients. By and large, the public no longer chooses to take their doctor's advice as the final word on certain health concerns. We are far more likely today to ask questions, seek second opinions, and research alternative treatments. The patient, rather than the doctor, is now the decision-maker when the patient's wellness is concerned.

What IS Modern Medicine Good For?

America's current "health" care system promotes drugs and surgery above all else – including prevention. Spending on medicines in America increased by double digits for a second year in 2015 and reached $425 billion. The first tragedy of this situation is that despite all that spending, America is still getting sicker and sicker. The second tragedy is that most of the illnesses for which we seek crisis care are completely preventable. Make no mistake: modern medicine still plays an important role in our healthcare system and the more open and receptive your primary care physician is to discuss your wellness care, the more of a partner role he or she can play in your ongoing health.

The modern view on health care places all health-related concepts and activities into three categories:

1. Self-care – this includes the choices you make every day about diet, exercise, stress management, and the like.

2. Health care – this is all of the things you seek help for in order to maintain good health, such as seeking wellness providers, getting educated on fitness and exercise, and taking part in wellness programs physicians are offering.

3. Crisis Care – this is the care we obtain when a disaster strikes; when we get sick or injured, and we go to the doctor or emergency room to help us fix what we cannot handle on our own.

Self-care and healthcare are intended to prevent the need for crisis care. However, choosing to stop smoking will not prevent you from getting into a car accident. There are sure-fire ways to prevent cancer, heart attacks, or other conditions but, of course, there are occurrences where serious illnesses, broken bones, failing organs are the rightful domain of crisis care.

A Crash Course in How to Get Well

Chances are there are about a hundred lifestyle choices you could improve upon. Here are a few simple suggestions to get you back on track:

- Get regular, moderate exercise (at least 30 minutes, three times a week)
- Stay well hydrated (Drink eight 8-ounce glasses of water a day)
- Eat mostly a plant-based, nutrient-dense diet
- Get adequate sleep (at least 7 hours/day)
- Quit smoking and any other drug habits

- Enjoy low alcohol intake (at the most, 5 drinks/week)
- Find healthy ways to deal with stress (exercise, yoga, stretching, meditation, prayer)
- Seek activities and people that boost your mood
- Bring aboard health care practitioners you trust to guide you, advise you, and provide treatments/therapies for your particular needs, health challenges, and health optimization goals.

In later chapters, we will dig into many of these topics in more detail. Suffice it to say that people tend to feel stressed and conflicted when making these lifestyle shifts. It's just so much easier to give in to our desires – to be lazy and not hit the gym; to order the cheeseburger because it's on the happy hour menu but the salad isn't; to quit smoking - "maybe next week."
All of those choices we make every day seem insignificant in the moment. But it all adds up. In ten, twenty, thirty years, will you regret your lifestyle choices? What it all comes down to is this – how can you improve your current level of functioning?

How to Choose Your Primary Doctor

In a word; <u>carefully</u>. I believe we could all use a great primary doctor on our wellness team. I also think that this PCP could be a chiropractor (we are trained to know when to refer out for help), a naturopath, an osteopath or a wellness minded medical doctor to name the most common. Granted, there are times that we may need the emergency room, but day-in-day-out health and wellness, sickness and disease, we need a great doc, one who is like-minded, very supportive and shares our health goals.

Despite the grim numbers that the field of medicine is putting up, there are fabulous MDs out there and they are getting easier and easier to find – especially with the World Wide Web. Here are some choice words you can put in your web browser to find the doc who'll support real healing.

- Alternative
- Complementary
- Integrative
- Natural
- Progressive
- Holistic

Word of mouth is always a great way to find a doctor too. Just ask around. Going to places of wellness and healing, like the local gyms or the nutrition and vitamin stores can be productive. Asking your massage therapist, chiropractor, acupuncturist or other practitioners can be extremely fruitful.

After you've narrowed it down to a few, check out the practitioner's website. Does it speak to you? Do you feel a connection? Read the testimonials on places like Google review (just "Google" the doctor's name), Yelp,

Angieslist.com, etc. How many stars does s/he have? What are the comments like?

Finally, call the doc's office and critique how you are handled by the staff. Now, I wouldn't necessarily judge the book by its cover, but you would get a sense of the team. The receptionist is the portal to the doctor. Chances are, you'll be communicating with this person just as much as the doctor. Let him or her know that you are looking for your next Primary Care Physician, have heard great things about this doctor and was wondering if s/he would be willing to do a "meet and greet" for maybe 5 or 10 minutes so you can get to know him/her. It's not unreasonable to ask this. You might be offered a phone discussion and, considering how busy we all are, I would think this to be an acceptable alternative to the in-person meeting. After all of that, it'll come down to a hunch – your gut feeling…trust it and go with it.

If you begin working with this practitioner and later determine that you made a wrong choice, FIRE him! Please, please, please keep in mind that we work for YOU, not the other way around. I've servred so many patients over the years who say things like; "Well, I've been with him for so long, I can't imagine leaving." Or, "I don't want to hurt her feelings". Or "My doctor's really nice, but he has no idea how to handle this."

My answer is always the same. "Why on earth do you keep him/her on your team?" It'd be like a pro football team keeping the "nice" quarterback in the starting lineup. If he's not getting the job done, MOVE ON! You wouldn't keep a painter employed who does a terrible job, slops the whole house up with paint and constantly shows up late, would you? Of course, you wouldn't. The business of YOUR health is what this is about and we only get one of these lives. If s/he's not cutting the mustard, move on!

Ok, time for me to move on too. In the next chapter, I'm really going to get into it by defining this "peripheral neuropathy" thing. Once we do that, I'll begin to unfold the blueprint for getting rid of it.

Chapter 4

What You Need to Know about Peripheral Neuropathy

Case Study

Sometimes patients come into my office with neuropathy that has gotten so bad they begin to lose their will to live. This story comes from a patient who said, "It was unbearable. Three months ago, I was begging my husband to take an axe, a saw or something and just cut my feet off." Her feet were burning, severely numb, tingling, and swollen. This was a severe case of neuropathy brought on by diabetes.

At the end of her program, she stated that she felt 95% better and our tests indicated an 80% improvement of the functioning of the nerves in the feet. "I have more energy; I can get up and do things whenever I want to. Three months ago, I couldn't do that because it was just so unbearable; me even standing on my feet. Now I'm walking and doing things around my house, and going places with my husband. I wanted him to just let me lay there and die. I've lost almost 30 pounds on this program and my diabetes numbers haven't been this good in probably a decade.

I have an appointment with my PCP coming up and I'm gonna rub it in [my doctor's] face because she told me there was nothing that could be done. She said I was gonna have to deal with it the rest of my life. I didn't think there was any hope out there until I found you guys. It's an amazing program. To all of you other diabetic neuropathy sufferers, do this: get off the sugars, get off the sodas and eat real food. You can reverse your neuropathy too!"

A Lesson in Neuroanatomy

Before diving into what is peripheral neuropathy, we'll need to lay out some anatomy or, rather *neuroanatomy*. It helps to break the term down and look at each individual word. **"Neuropathy"** means damage to nerves. **"Peripheral"** refers to the peripheral nervous system – that's all of the nerves in your body that radiate out from your spinal cord and brain.

Let's first talk about the Central Nervous System (CNS). Essentially this consists of the brain and the spinal cord. We often call the CNS our "onboard computer" – the organ that controls the whole body.

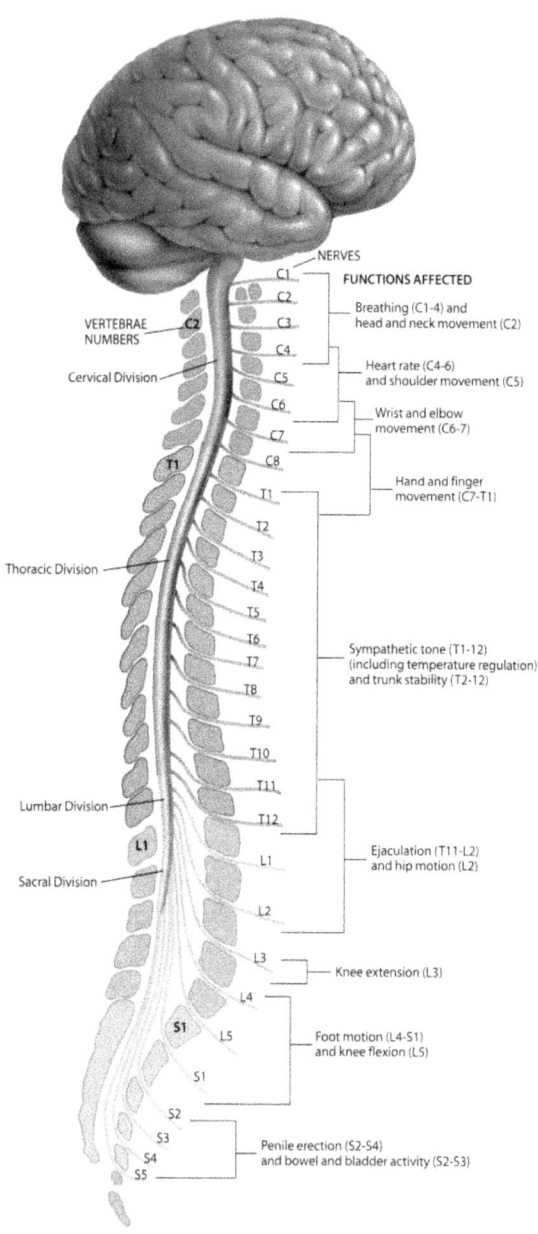

NERVES

FUNCTIONS AFFECTED

C1
C2
C3
Breathing (C1-4) and
head and neck movement (C2)
C4
C5
Heart rate (C4-6)
and shoulder movement (C5)
C6
Wrist and elbow
movement (C6-7)
C7
C8
Hand and finger
movement (C7-T1)
T1
T2
T3
T4
T5
T6
T7
Sympathetic tone (T1-12)
(including temperature regulation)
and trunk stability (T2-12)
T8
T9
T10
T11
T12
Ejaculation (T11-L2)
and hip motion (L2)
L1
L2
L3
Knee extension (L3)
L4
L5
Foot motion (L4-S1)
and knee flexion (L5)
S1
S2
S3
Penile erection (S2-S4)
S4
and bowel and bladder activity (S2-S3)
S5

VERTEBRAE
NUMBERS   **C2**

Cervical Division

T1

Thoracic Division

Lumbar Division   **L1**

Sacral Division

S1

Now, the Peripheral Nervous System (PNS) consists of all the nerves that leave either the brain or the spinal cord – it is "peripheral" to the Central Nervous System. Most neuropathies refer to the nerves that exit the spinal cord and go down to the arms, hands and fingers or down to the legs, feet and toes.

The diagram shows the main peripheral nerves that travel down the arms and legs.

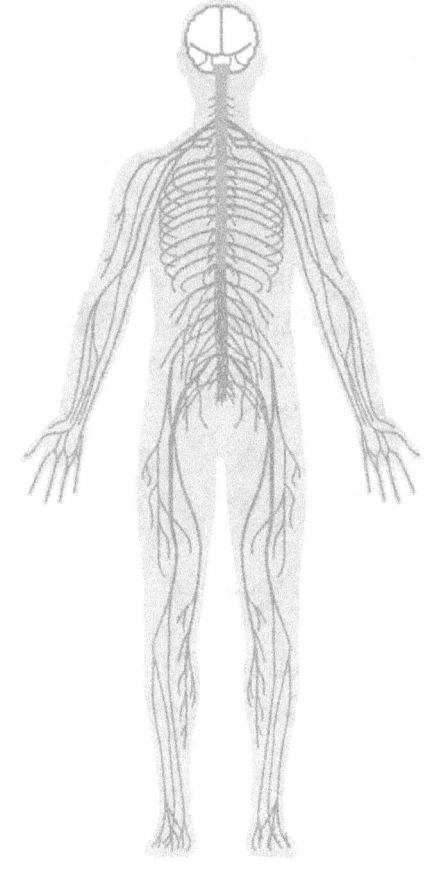

Common Symptoms of Peripheral Neuropathy:

There are so many different things you can feel when your nerves begin to die off or have already died, but here are the most common ones I hear about:

- burning
- hypersensitivity of the extremities
- sharp, stabbing pains
- tingling
- numbness
- inability to feel heat or cold
- feet or hands always feel hot or cold
- achiness, tightness, and/or swelling in the extremities
- "weird" sensations like, ants crawling around, socks feeling like they are bunched up, a feeling like there is a piece of cardboard stuck to the bottom of the feet
- inability to grasp small items like needles, pens or pencils, buttons
- balance problems
- weakness
- Restless Leg Syndrome

Next, we need to discuss the Autonomic Nervous System (ANS) because it is a part of the PNS.

There are two parts to the ANS – the Sympathetic and the Parasympathetic Nervous System. Basically, the

Parasympathetic Nervous System calms down our internal organs and the Sympathetic Nervous System speeds them up. It's the Rest and Recuperation vs. the Flight or Fight systems. Both are necessary to our survival. Here's what is so important about the ANS as it relates to Peripheral Neuropathy.

Possible Symptoms of Peripheral Neuropathy as it Relates to the ANS:

- High or low blood pressure
- Asthma, COPD, lung issues
- Acid reflux, gastroparesis
- Irritable bowel syndrome, constipation, diarrhea
- Pre-diabetes / diabetes
- Incontinence (loss of bowel and/or bladder control)
- Erectile dysfunction

Other Symptoms of Peripheral Neuropathy

Neuropathy of the small fiber nerves reduces sensation and can cause the patient not to be able to feel cuts, burns, punctures, or blisters on the skin. Reduced sensation in the feet can cause car accidents when people fail to sense whether they are pressing the gas pedal or the brake or they may not be able to regulate the pressure they apply to a pedal.

Neuropathy in the legs can cause loss of balance and coordination. This type of neuropathy causes thousands of falls every year. A fall puts the patient at risk for hip fractures, head traumas, and other serious injuries, which is the number one cause of death in senior citizens.

What Causes Peripheral Neuropathy?

Instead of delving into the hundreds of specific causes for peripheral neuropathy, we will break them down into six general categories.

1. **Circulation related peripheral neuropathy** is most often experienced by people with diabetes, but anyone with reduced blood circulation is at risk. When the small blood vessels surrounding the nerves die off, the nerves are deprived of nourishment and will also eventually die. It is the damaged nerves that are the source of pain, numbness and tingling. Over 50% of diabetics develop some form of neuropathy (Mayo Clinic). Peripheral neuropathy is also the top cause of amputations for diabetics.

2. **Toxicity related peripheral neuropathy** can be caused by any sort of exposure to toxins. The three causes we typically focus on are chemotherapy drugs, statin drugs and other medications.

   a. **Chemotherapy-induced peripheral neuropathy** is a side effect reported by many cancer patients who have received chemotherapy. Some chemotherapy drugs like Cisplatin, Vincristine, Paclitaxel, Etoposide, Teniposide and others are more likely to cause neuropathy than others. Patients who are on a more frequent treatment schedule are also more likely to experience neuropathy. Other drugs used to treat cancer such as Thalidomide and Interferon can also cause peripheral neuropathy.

b. **Statin-induced peripheral neuropathy** is caused by the use of drugs that doctors prescribe to reduce fats, including triglycerides and cholesterol, in the blood. Instead of prescribing changes in diet and exercise habits to fix the root cause of the cholesterol problem, it is far easier (and more profitable) for a doctor to prescribe a Statin medication. Check your medicine cabinet for any of these drugs and ask your doctor if this drug is possibly causing your neuropathy; Atorvastatin, Fluvastatin, Lovastatin, Pitavastatin, Pravastatin, Rosuvastatin and Simvastatin. Basically, if the drug name ends in "statin", it could be causing peripheral nerve damage. The most common symptoms of statin-induced neuropathy are muscle pain, cramping and weakness. Further, the damage may persist even after statin use is halted, meaning these drugs may cause permanent muscle damage.

c. **Other Medications**. You may not believe this but here are some other drugs that may cause peripheral neuropathy:
   1. Anti-alcohol drugs (Disulfiram)
   2. Anticonvulsants (Phenytoin / Dilantin®, Gabapentin)
   3. Heart or blood pressure medications (Amiodarone, Hydralazine, Perhexiline)
   4. Antibiotics (Metronidazole, Flagyl®, Cipro®, Levaquin®, Nitrofurantoin, Isoniazid, Dapsone)

a. **Alcohol;** Abuse of alcohol can lead to a B vitamin deficiency that, in turn, can lead to peripheral neuropathy.

2. **Trauma induced peripheral neuropathy** is caused by events like car accidents, falls, or athletic injuries. Any of these events can cause damage to the peripheral nerves. Wearing a cast, walking with crutches or frequent repetitive motions can also damage nerves.

3. **Spinal Causes.** Many of the patients who consult with me for their neuropathy have already been tested by MRI, CT scans, X-rays and/or EMG's. These tests are specifically designed to rule out problems in the spine itself. Designed to protect the spinal cord and the exiting spinal nerve roots (that travel down the arms and legs), problems often develop from birth or traumas throughout life. Conditions like Scoliosis, Degenerative Arthritis, Bulging disc, Osteoporosis, old spinal fractures and stenosis to name just a few of the many problems that can irritate those peripheral nerves and cause neuropathy.

4. **Other Causes.** As mentioned, there are over 100 different causes of peripheral neuropathy, and some of them won't fit neatly into the top 4 categories. Conditions in this category include (but are not limited to): Multiple Sclerosis, Lou Gehrig's disease (ALS), Agent Orange induced neuropathy, mold poisoning, stroke, paralysis, autoimmune diseases, transverse myelitis, heavy metal poisoning, vitamin deficiencies, anemia, and many others.

5. **Idiopathic peripheral neuropathy.** This basically means that we do not know the cause of the neuropathy.

One important fact to realize is that regardless of the cause of peripheral neuropathy, the damage is the same under a microscope. The techniques for rebuilding the nerves do not change. We'll talk about that in the next chapter.

Chapter 5

How Do We Treat Peripheral Neuropathy?

Case Study

I recall a case a while back when an older patient came in with horrible neuropathy in both his feet and hands – tingling, numbness and pain all bundled up together 24/7. Do you know all the boxes on a doctor's new patient paperwork with all the possible symptoms one could have? Well, he had just about ALL of them checked off. I mean this poor man was in some serious pain.

Turns out he was a soldier during Vietnam. He did a lot of jumping out of planes and, at one point, for a period of about a year, his job was to project Agent Orange out of the airplane as it flew over enemy territory. He explained to me that, at the time, no one knew of the damaging effects of this very toxic chemical. So that's why they gave all the men bandanas to wear over their faces. Nothing more than a cloth bandana. Not a mask with fresh oxygen, no eye or any skin protection at all -just a bandana.

Well, NOW we know that Agent Orange is VERY toxic to humans and one of its terrible afflictions is *peripheral neuropathy. When I ran the neuropathy testing, he had 99% loss of the nerves in both feet and 80% loss in the hands. Sadly, I had to break it to this veteran who served our country bravely and proudly that the natural therapies used in our program would **NOT** realistically return his feet to normal, but we still had a "fair" chance on his hands. Since his feet were by far the most irritating for him, he decided **NOT** to start any care. It was sad for me to see him walk out the door because I know for sure I could have helped him significantly ten years ago.*

The moral of the story? Don't wait until your neuropathy is too far advanced. This is a progressive condition that just keeps getting worse and worse.

So, how DO we treat peripheral neuropathy...now THAT is the question, right? That's why you picked up this book in the first place. What I'm about ready to say is probably going to shock you, but you need to hear it. This is the crux of the entire program – the crème de la crème. This next statement is why we are able to appreciate an 85% success rate when doctors and Western medicine are failing miserably. OK – here we go:

We do NOT treat peripheral neuropathy at all! "What?" you say. "If you don't treat it, then how come you wrote a book on it?" The fact is that neither I, nor your PCP, nor the best neurologist has a single clue on how to actually fix a nerve that is dying in your feet or hands (let alone thousands of nerves that are shot). We really don't, but the great news is that your body actually does.

That is also the incredibly uplifting news. Yes, the reason we get such amazing results with a condition that is supposedly "impossible" to cure is that we tap into the most valuable tool known to (wo)man. We have - already built into us - the ability to self-heal! Whether you want to say it was "God given" or "nature derived" or just a part of the survival mechanism, we are self-healers. D.D. Palmer, the founder of chiropractic, called it "Innate Intelligence" which means that we have an inborn intelligence that knows how to run our body, and that includes healing it when it is injured or sick. Whatever you want to call it, it's BIG!

Let's break it down to a simple scenario. Let's say that you leave your house for an extended vacation – say four weeks. You shut the house down, turn the AC off, close the blinds, lock up and leave. When you return four weeks later and open the blinds, you discover that all of your house plants are in serious trouble. Most are either dead or look that way.

What would be your first instinct? You'd probably be upset, but I'm sure you'd grab the watering can and water them! Next, you might move them a little closer to the windows, or if it's nice enough, bring them to the outside for better sun exposure. To help out, you may even offer them a little soil amendment with some fertilizer or Miracle-Gro®.

What would you do next? Most likely? **NOTHING**. You'd get out of the way and let nature take its course, realizing that, as long as the plant isn't completely dead, it'll come back, right? Well, that is our exact method, but we do it the human way. We give your body what it needs and take away what is hurting it. It's so dang simple I really don't understand why more physicians and "experts" don't "get" this concept. Why is neuropathy such a head scratcher? Boggles my mind.

Medical doctors routinely tell their patients that nerves cannot regenerate themselves, but it's simply not true! Most of our patients are told, "There is nothing that can be done for peripheral neuropathy." Or "You need to learn to live with it," or "You're just getting older."

Regardless of the naysayers, for the majority of peripheral neuropathy cases, <u>reversing peripheral neuropathy is not impossible</u>. This is why I titled the book *Reversing Peripheral Neuropathy: Making the Impossible Possible.* It does take work though. Several treatments have been proven to stimulate the growth of the nerve endings and the blood vessels that nourish them.

If a treatable underlying condition causes the symptoms, it is almost always possible to reverse your neuropathy. While medications can reduce the pain associated with peripheral neuropathy, painkillers do nothing to repair or reverse the damage to the nerves and blood vessels. And what about numbness? There is no drug to cover up the symptom of numbness or tingling – it doesn't even exist. Getting to the root cause of the neuropathy and taking steps to reverse the damage is the only effective and long-lasting method of treatment. Bottom line? You will never, ever be able to medicate yourself out of peripheral neuropathy.

The end goal in treating neuropathy is to remove blockages so that the nerves can function properly and send and receive messages to and from the brain. The best way to achieve this is with a comprehensive treatment plan. That's why we use several methods concurrently to treat our peripheral neuropathy patients. At our clinic, peripheral neuropathy appointments last about 45 minutes rather than the standard 10-15-minute visit with the MD.

Toronto Clinical Scoring System

Before I get into how we treat neuropathy, I'll need to go over how it is diagnosed. Expensive studies like EMG (Electromyography), NCV (Nerve Conduction Velocity), MRI (Magnetic Resonance Imaging), X-ray and others can be helpful but the Toronto Clinical Scoring System (TCSS) is a much easier and less invasive way to figure out how bad those nerves have been damaged. Additionally it can be used to check for progress and treatment outcomes. The TCSS has been found to be a valid and reliable tool used for the diagnosis and staging of diabetic and all other types of sensorimotor polyneuropathy.

Peripheral Neuropathy Treatment Options

Below is a partial list of the treatments that we have found to be extremely helpful for our neuropathy cases. As science continually changes and our understanding of neuropathy increases, more and better treatments are added and old ones are subtracted or replaced. Let's start with the list, in no particular order, and in the following chapters we'll dig a bit deeper into how they work.

Nutrition – This one should start at the top of all doctor's treatments no matter what the condition. Committing to dietary changes that reduce inflammation in the body can make a tremendous difference in reversing peripheral neuropathy. An anti-inflammatory diet promotes foods that inhibit the damaging effect of inflammation (meats, vegetables, fruits, nuts, and seeds) and limits the intake of foods that promote inflammation (sugars, starches, omega-6 foods, alcohol, and smoking). (See Chapter 6)

Supplements – Theoretically, we should be able to get all that we need to survive and thrive from a good, clean diet. In this day and age, with an agricultural industry that is more interested in making a quick buck (billions of bucks, actually), a lot of shortcuts are taken, and we, therefore, need to supplement our diet. There are many supplements that the modern human should take to fill in the gaps left by our food supply, but for this book, I'll focus on those we prescribe in most cases for neuropathy. Basically, we use supplements that decrease inflammation and increase nitric oxide. (See Chapter 6)

Low-Level Light Therapy (LLLT) – LLLT uses low-power lasers or infrared light-emitting diodes to promote artery growth, reduce pain, improve immune response, accelerate healing of wounds and fractures, increase collagen and DNA production, and promote fibroblast activity. Among other functions LLLT stimulates the release of the Nobel Prize winning molecule called nitric oxide. (See Chapter 7)

Electrotherapy – We use an FDA approved tool called The ReBuilder® in our clinic. It uses low frequency, electrical stimulation to improve and normalize deficits in nerve conduction velocity. The ReBuilder System® is trusted by all five Cancer Treatment Centers of America® locations to alleviate chemotherapy-induced peripheral neuropathy. I figure if it's working for them, why wouldn't it work for us? And it does! We've been successfully using it since 2010. (See Chapter 8)

Brain-Based Therapy (BBT) – BBT allows signals to flow between the brain, spinal cord, and nerves. Since BBT promotes nervous system function, it should be considered an integral part of any peripheral neuropathy treatment plan. The receptors in the hands and feet are connected to nerves which travel all the way up to the brain where their signals are interpreted. A comprehensive neuropathy program must include therapies and treatments that include improving the function of the brain. (See Chapter 9)

Vibration Therapy – Vibration therapy increases balance and mobility, bone density, and range of motion. It also increases blood flow by 15 times. During vibration therapy, patients sit or stand on a vibrating platform that causes their muscles to contract, increase circulation, as well as nerve stimulation. (See Chapter 10)

Soft Tissue Therapy – Hand-held soft tissue machines are used to massage the tissue surrounding the areas affected by peripheral neuropathy. Soft tissue therapy targets injured muscles and soft tissue. Light and deep pressure manual therapies, joint mobilization, Trigenics®, stretching and trigger point techniques are used to promote the restoration of function, improved circulation, and breaking down scar tissue. (See Chapter 11)

Spinal Decompression – When peripheral neuropathy has resulted from an accident or injury that led to compressed discs or vertebrae, spinal decompression can provide relief. It is a technique that uses specific traction to take the pressure off the discs and allows the them to move back into place. It also stimulates blood flow, which produces a healing response. (See Chapter 12)

Exercise – Time and time again exercise proves itself in the research to help with just about every ailment known to man, but here's the conundrum with peripheral neuropathy and exercise. It hurts too darn much to do it. Check out chapter 13 where I go over how to return to exercise in a safe and pain-free way.

What Else Is There?

There are many layers that make up a condition like neuropathy. Many of those are discussed in this book – neurological, skeletal, muscular and vascular – but let's not forget the others that may sometimes be difficult to measure and "treat." Psychological, emotional and even spiritual layers are almost always there as well. Are you a positive thinker, or is that glass always half empty? Do you *believe* that your neuropathy can be helped or are you completely hopeless? Do you think that ALL of the healing should come in a bottle or surgery or do you ponder that the body has an inborn wisdom that is engineered to self-heal?

In my opinion, all of the fancy equipment and gadgets that we use are of little value if a patient is completely hopeless. Sometimes we'll need to spend more time on beliefs before we start the healing process. While we provide our patients with the resources to make the right choices for themselves, it is solely up to you as to how closely you follow these guidelines. In the next few chapters, I'll be diving deeper into the treatments listed above.

Are you ready to heal? Are you sick and tired of being sick and tired? Has the time come to get your life back? If the answer is yes, then turn to the next page!

Chapter 6

Nutrition and Supplementation

Case Study

Bill M. had a complex case of Diabetic Neuropathy that presented as tingling, numbness, and pain in his hands and feet. His feet were so painful that he had difficulty standing for any period of time. The sensitivity in his hands was so severe that he was barely able to grip or turn a page in a book. He was an avid reader and loved to play golf, but had to give up these two hobbies. Like many of my neuropathy patients, Bill had diabetes and was taking gabapentin, along with 8 other medications. After 2 months of care, Bill came into the office and told us he had woken up the morning before and said, "Jeez, my feet feel good today".

At the end of his care program, Bill left us with this glowing testimonial: "I was on metformin and gabapentin for a year; they didn't seem to do anything. Thanks to your program, it has made a big difference. I started out with diabetes and then reversed it with your diet and supplement recommendations. I am learning to eat the right foods, instead of everything the government tells us is so great for us. Now I have come to the point where I am getting some nerve endings renewed. I have a better sense of feeling in my hands and feet. I can walk better, I can walk further and I've lost 40 lbs., and it has given me a new lease on life. "

Oh, the last time I saw Bill, he had just golfed 18 holes…and he can flip the pages in his favorite books. He was completely off metformin and gabapentin. On his final re-evaluation, he stated that he felt 60-70% better and on our nerve testing his hands had improved by 40% and feet by over 50%. Not bad for two "impossible" to reverse conditions like diabetes and neuropathy, huh?

As I stated earlier, nutrition is the place where most treatment programs should start.

Skipping this step with neuropathy is like building a house on sand. It won't work. You have got to form a solid foundation from which health can build upon. Oh, by the way, "health" is what we are going for in my "Reversing Neuropathy Program." Healing your nerves is going to be a "side effect" of getting you healthy. You must understand this point.

Often, in my report of findings appointment where I'm giving my recommendations, I'll stop right after I've laid out my nutritional plan and ask the patient a simple question. "Ms. Jones, do you think you can follow these dietary recommendations? Because if you can't, we should stop right here, shake hands and agree to be friends." Seriously, I tell them, "it's that important." If they can't give me their word that they'll try their best for at least 30 days, then I don't even bother with explaining all of the fancy equipment we use to support and speed the healing of the nerves.

Nutrition in a Nutshell

We have to decrease the metabolic inflammation in those nerve pathways, and it's very manageable to do. The way that we correct those is by recommending a clean, healthy, anti-inflammatory diet. Here are the basics of this diet: No sugar, no dairy, no refined grains like wheat and no alcohol. Most patients at this point are like: **"YIKES! WHAT CAN I EAT?!"**This is where I get the raised eyebrows, frowns, and blank stares. For most, I've just taken away a large portion of their daily foods and they are imagining that they'll need to be starving for the next 30 days. Well, let's talk about what's left to eat. People, what you're left with is REAL FOOD! It's what humans are supposed to be eating for your nerve's sake!

Foods like:
- beef (yes, even steak)
- chicken
- turkey
- pork (yes, even bacon)
- fish
- venison
- bison
- eggs
- vegetables (and lots of them)

- fruits
- nuts (and nut butter)
- seeds (and seed butter)
- almond, coconut, hemp milk
- herbal and green teas
- water
- lots more too

There's plenty of food to eat; we're just taking away all the crap, ok? This is not a calorie restricted diet, and you will never be hungry on it. For my patients, we have a ton of recipes and food shopping lists too (make sure to check out the companion cookbook to this book). In case you are wondering, this is similar to "The Paleo Diet." Look it up on the internet. The bestselling book by Loren Cordain, Ph.D. is entitled simply; *The Paleo Diet.* I'd strongly recommend getting the book. It's a reference book with recipes and explanations. Listen, this diet is easy to follow. You just have to decide if you're going to suck it up and go for it, or not.

Now, the benefits of this diet are enormous.
The first thing is that it's going to decrease inflammation in your entire body– especially those nerve-endings in the feet and hands. So, I expect you will start noticing differences in how you feel, very quickly – now it's different for every patient, but somewhere within in the first week to the third week you're going to notice that you're feeling a lot better.

The second thing is this: your blood sugar, your blood pressure, your cholesterol, your triglycerides, and other blood markers that your doctor is measuring and probably medicating for are going to be healthier than they've been in a long time. These are very significant changes happening in a very short period of time.

The next thing you'll notice is energy; and I mean a lot of it. I'm not talking about the artificial energy you've been accustomed to from sodas and coffee, I mean REAL, organic, human-made ENERGY! Those highs and lows you now feel throughout the day? You might as well put that behind you. It's part of your history. You'll be blown away at how much more energy you're going to have and how level it'll be throughout your day. Napping? Thing of the past. Gone. You just won't need them anymore. You won't even feel the need for them. It's remarkable how dang fast your body is going to be at healing itself.

And the last thing is, you might drop five to ten pounds within that first month, ok? And that's just an added bonus of getting healthier.

What's so bad about wheat?

Ok, I get this one all the time, so I might as well cover it right now. Here are questions and statements I get:

- "I thought that whole grain wheat is supposed to be healthy for me."

- "What about Ezekiel bread or sprouted wheat…aren't those good for me?"
- "What about rye bread? Is that ok?"

Wheat is a double-edged sword. Remember from chapter two when I went over the glycemic index (GI)? The index that tells us how fast certain foods convert into blood sugar (glucose). Glucose itself is assigned the value of 100, and all other foods are compared to it. So, the higher the number, the faster the food converts into blood sugar. Too much blood sugar for too long of a period (a lifetime for most of us), burns out the pancreas from combating this never-ending onslaught of sugar.

Well, too much sugar in the blood KILLS NERVES, especially the nerve endings (as a side note, it kills other organs too, like the kidneys, retina in the eye and even the brain itself). When you finally destroy your pancreas, and it poops out in its ability to release insulin, we call that "Diabetes Type 2". On your way to diabetes you are killing nerves too, so just because you don't (yet) have it, if you are not regulating blood sugars well enough, you ARE KILLING NERVES, so STOP IT!

Whoops, I got a little sidetracked there. Lemme step off the soap box and get back to wheat. So, on your plate, that piece of toast that you had for breakfast converted into glucose in your blood FASTER than if you just ate a bunch of table sugar. Did you get that? Whole wheat bread's glycemic index is 69, and that of table sugar is 65. Bottom line? It's not what's *on* your plate that matters; it's what your body *does* with what's on your plate that matters. You might as well be taking a blow torch to your nerves in your feet and hands because that's pretty much what you are doing.

Consider this: how many teaspoons of sugar are in two slices of supposedly healthy multi-grain bread? Well, let's see, there are 18 grams of non fiber carbohydrates per slice x 2 equals 36 grams. Divide that by 4 and you get 9 grams of sugar. Yes, you read that right, after your body breaks down that wheat you have just eaten the equivalent of nine (9) teaspoons of sugar! Now how many teaspoons of sugar are in that very sweet tasting Snickers bar? 8.5 teaspoons of sugar. So, two thin slices of whole wheat bread have more sugar than a Snickers bar. Hey, don't get me wrong here. I'm not saying that a Snickers bar is healthy, ok? This is just "food for thought."

On the other edge of the wheat sword is the gluten riddle. I know you've heard of gluten. How could you not in this day and age when so many items are marketed and made gluten-free. Seems like everywhere you turn there's "gluten-free". You can even get Oreo cookies gluten-free! Jeez, Louise. I guess the term "gluten-free" sells, huh?

Anyway, it turns out this gluten thing is not another phase or fad. According to The National Foundation

Brian Prax

for Celiac Awareness, only 1% of Americans have Celiac Disease, which means they are ALLERGIC to the gluten protein in wheat, rye, and barley and they need to avoid it like the plague because, in time, it'll kill them. On the other hand, it is estimated that 18 million Americans may have "Non-Celiac Gluten Sensitivity" (NCGS). They won't die from gluten but they will certainly be uncomfortable.

Some symptoms include:
- bloating and gassy especially right after eating gluten
- diarrhea, constipation and smelly feces
- abdominal pain
- depression and anxiety
- ADHD/ADD
- brain fog
- autoimmune disease
- low immunity
- dental issues
- unexplained weight loss or weight gain
- migraine (and other) headaches
- skin problems (eczema, rashes, itchy blisters, pimples)
- hormonal imbalance
- joint and muscle aches
- numbness or tingling in the arms and legs
- extreme fatigue

So, considering the double-edged sword of wheat, I recommend that all of my peripheral neuropathy patients to stop eating it…100%. You can't just cut back on it; you must stop it completely. After 30 days, if you want to try it out, you can do so, but take stock of how you are feeling before doing so and then how you feel after. If you have any of the symptoms listed above, you, too, may be gluten sensitive or perhaps you could have Celiac Disease. At that point, you'll have a decision to make. Have your cake and suffer or not have your cake and live your life way more comfortably. By the way, if you want a great book to read on the subject, you should read *"Wheat Belly,"* by cardiologist William Davis, MD.

Dairy, Dairy, so Contrary

Dairy products include food items such as yogurt, cheese, butter and, of course, milk. They are specifically designed for the cow's (or goat's) infants –not humans. I know, I know, you grew up drinking milk and eating cheese and yogurt and so did I. Be aware that the American Dairy Association advertises like crazy to get us to buy into the lie that cow's milk is good for humans.

Totally not true. Not only is it inflammatory for us, but it's been so altered from its normal state, it's not even the same food it was when it first came out of the udder. Remember milk back in the 50s and 60s when it was delivered by the milkman in glass containers?

Remember also how the cream floated to the top and your mom (or you) used that cream for making butter, putting in your coffee and other things? It also had such a short shelf life it would last maybe five days if you got it into the icebox quick enough, right? Well, that's not long enough for sales, you know so, nowadays, milk is significantly altered. Some, if not all the fat is removed, then it is pasteurized, homogenized and bastardized. They add vitamin D to it and then ship it out in trucks hundreds of miles from the farm.

Oh, and here's another thing with milk – calcium. Doesn't, "Milk do a body good?" Well, that's what they tell us over and over again, correct? So, let me tell you the other half of the story. The part that they don't want you to know. They say that milk is an excellent source of calcium and that is true, but, just like in the wheat example, it's not what's in your glass that matters, instead, it's what your body *does* with what's in your glass. Just read this excerpt from www.saveourbones.com and decide for yourself.

> "Like all animal protein, milk acidifies the body pH which in turn triggers a biological correction. You see, calcium is an excellent acid neutralizer and the biggest storage of calcium in the body is (you guessed it) in the bones. So the very same calcium that our bones need to stay strong is utilized to neutralize the acidifying effect of milk. Once calcium is pulled out of the bones, it leaves the body via the urine so that

the surprising net result after this is an actual calcium deficit.

Knowing this, you'll understand why statistics show that countries with the lowest consumption of dairy products also have the lowest fracture incidence in their population."

In addition to that, you may also be lactose (or other milk property) intolerant. You likely know someone who has lactose intolerance and they just need to flat out avoid it. It makes them very uncomfortable to eat it. The reality is that you, too, may be intolerant to it as well and just not know it. How will you know? It's simple: you'd either pay for an expensive blood test or fast from it for at least 30 days. Then, add it back in and see how you feel. Go ahead, give it a try. I promise you won't die and your bones won't turn to dust in a month's time!

Does milk really do a body good? Yes, in a calf's body, but not your body. You are human, and you only needed human milk for the first year or so; it's time to grow out of it! We are the only species on the planet that drinks the milk of another species. Isn't it a bit weird to think about a kangaroo drinking the milk from a zebra? Besides, it's certainly not good for your nerves. To be accepted into our neuropathy program, our patients have to commit to at least a 30 day fast of dairy.

Drink Up

Water makes up 70% of planet earth and amazingly about the same amount in the human body. I'd say it's the most forgotten yet important molecule in the healing world. It is estimated that up to 75% of Americans are chronically dehydrated. It is needed in just about all of the chemical reactions that occur in the body and it also:

- regulates your body temperature
- protects the brain and spinal cord by acting as a cushion
- lubricates your joints
- is crucial in the excretion and detoxification processes
- aids in digestion

Not to mention the obvious. Without it, we die! We can live without food for up to 3 weeks, maybe longer, in the ideal situation but, in the BEST scenario, we can make it only about a week without water.

Here's something to keep in mind when trying to figure out how much to drink. Obviously, it depends on many factors:

- how much you weigh
- the temperature
- being in direct sunlight
- vigorous exercise
- And more

Keep in mind that we lose water quickly when we are sick, have diarrhea or are vomiting. They say that we are supposed to drink eight 8-ounce glasses of water per day —that nearly fills up a 2-liter bottle. Keep in mind that we get water from the foods we eat too. Watermelon, cantaloupe, and strawberries have up to 92% water in them, but did you know that vegetables like zucchini, cauliflower and spinach have a ton of water in them too? Even carrots have 87% water in them. So, getting your 4-5 servings of veggies and fruits a day adds to your overall water consumption.

The ole 8-glasses a day is a great rule of thumb, but here's a better one if you don't like counting. LISTEN TO YOUR BODY! Try NEVER to let it get thirsty. When you are thirsty, you are behind! Hurry and drink some water or eat a carrot.

One of the strategies I use is to drink two large glasses of water first thing when I wake up. I'm usually thirsty anyway, and it's easy to do. Each of the pint glasses I use contains 16 ounces of water, so that gets me a great head start. I'm already at four of my eight glasses – half way there! My green tea later in the morning accounts for another one, and I'm off and running! Oh, of course, when I have run, swam or biked (or some other exercise), I need to add more water, right?

What about Juice, Gatorade®, Diet Sodas and Sweet Tea?

Ok, I thought I'd have to cover this at some point, so here goes. Humans are made to drink one thing…WATER! All the other stuff is, generally, NOT GOOD FOR US.

Juice – WAY TOO MUCH SUGAR. When you remove all of the fiber what you're left with is sugar water – BAD for you and definitely BAD for your nerves. Yeah, it has high levels of Vitamin C, but all that sugar? BAD, BAD, BAD. Here's what the bestselling author, Dr. Permutter (he's a neurologist who wrote *Grain Brain* – this is an excellent book by the way) has to say on the subject.[22]

> "The reality of the situation is that yes, a glass of orange juice does indeed contain some vitamin C, but that fact hardly outweighs the fact that O.J. is just loaded with sugar. A single 12-ounce glass of O.J. contains an incredible 9 teaspoons of sugar, about the same as a 12 ounce can of Coke! This equates to 36 grams of carbs, about half of what you should consume in a day."

---

[22]http://www.drperlmutter.com/about/grain-brain-by-david-perlmutter

Here's my quick answer to **Gatorade®** and other sports drinks. JUNK! The glycemic index of this beverage that is sold as a healthy alternative to sodas is a whopping 89! Enough said! Stay away, unless you are exercising VIGOROUSLY for OVER an hour – then MAYBE consume it. What's better for getting those electrolytes? Coconut water – try it out.

Diet sodas are HORRIBLE. They're even worse than the dang regular sodas, not that I'm saying regular sodas are good for you. All of them contain dubious, man-made chemical sweeteners that have an unproven track record. Lots of studies point to the possibility of the carcinogenic properties of these artificial sweeteners. Carcinogenic means CANCER – BAD stuff!

Research further suggests that these chemicals can throw off your body's natural metabolic processes. Disrupting these processes could cause your body to store fat instead of burning it, and may <u>increase</u> your risks for diabetes and heart disease. And if that wasn't enough, still more research shows that those who drink diet sodas on a regular basis consume more calories, which in turn adds more weight. Get them out of your refrigerator now. Don't even give them to your worst enemy.

Here in the south, it is customary to drink a lot of **sweet tea**, but, bottom line, sweet tea has too much sugar in it. I don't mind the "tea" part of it, but it's the "sweet" part that's not good for us. Try adding stevia (a natural sweetener) to your tea or, better yet, try and get used to your tea without anything added…well, I'd be fine with a squirt of lemon, ok?

I have the same exact recommendations for **coffee**. Drink it black if you can, or try adding a little bit of stevia if you must. For "cream" try some coconut creamer or other alternative creamer but, truth be told, none of those are really that good for us either.

Here's another thing about coffee. It's best to go with organic coffee as the countries that grow the beans use suspicious chemicals. Organic does not cost that much more, but it's always best to get food as clean and natural as possible and coffee is one of those foods that is important enough to go organic.

Oh, and we all know that coffee has the somewhat controversial chemical, caffeine, in it. This is similar to red wine (containing resveratrol) which has shown to be beneficial to the heart; I'd suggest keeping it in moderation. How about a cup of coffee a day…A CUP, OK? That does not mean a Venti, Caramel Macchiato, Skim, Extra Shot, Extra Hot, Extra Whip, Sugar-free, either – capiche?

To Supplement or Not to Supplement, That is the Question.

Eating a well-balanced diet *should* provide all of the essential nutrients, vitamins, enzymes, probiotics, minerals, and trace minerals for us, right? Well, this may have been true before the First World War and certainly in Jesus' time, but nowadays, in the modern world, when we dump oil and chemical based fertilizers on our soil – it's not going to happen.

You see, after WWI we had all of this petroleum just sitting around in abundance (that's why gas was just $0.20/gallon) and we wondered what we could do with it. Well, scientists also had to grapple with the dust bowl which resulted from farmers over farming the soils in the middle of America. Combine that with droughts, dust clouds were known to blow as far as the East Coast. We were left with one hundred million acres of soil that would barely grow a weed. Scientists figured out that plants need 3 basic elements – nitrogen, phosphorus and potassium, in order to grow. It turns out that synthetic fertilizers could supply those nutrients in large and cheap amounts.

The modern scientist knows that while a plant can *survive* on those three elements, the human needs to eat plants (and the animals that eat those plants) that are *organically* grown, which will supply all of the elements, minerals and nutrients needed to *thrive*. Having said all that, it is my belief, that in our modern, over-farmed worlds, we must supplement, so let's turn the discussion to that puzzle.

Centrum One a Day®, Centrum Silver® and the like are the most prescribed and recommended supplements in the U.S. of A. It's no wonder when one realizes that the pharmaceutical giant Pfizer is the manufacturer of Centrum® products. With the same access to doctors across America, reps dole out Centrum® like Pez® candy and doctors then hand out these vitamins to their patients.

But how good are Centrum® and other non-food based vitamins for us? In short – not at all. You may as well be swallowing pebbles one time a day because they are basically chemical cocktails that are made with some of the lowest grade vitamins and minerals known to scientists. Absorbability is the name of the game when it comes to vitamins. Like bread, it's not what's in the supplement that matters; it's what your body is able to DO with the supplement that matters. So, if bread is converted into sugar by the body, what is Centrum® and other chemical based tablets converted into? Answer: Nothing. Your body poops them right out. They are so non-absorbable your body doesn't even break them down in order to digest them. Basically, they are a colossal waste of money.

There are so many other better choices out there that I'd recommend, and whichever you choose, it needs to be "whole food" based. Like the name implies "whole food" means that, instead of nasty chemicals that are made in a lab somewhere, these vitamins are derived from foods that you can actually buy in a grocery store. Organic foods like spirulina, beet, broccoli, kale, spinach, blackberry, blueberry, carrot, cranberry, etc. Your body recognizes these as foods and absorbs them much, much better than the chemicals. Some of my favorite brands in no particular order are; Rainbow Light®, New Chapter®, Garden of Life® and Standard Process®.

When it comes to supplementing with vitamins and minerals, you get what you pay for and I'd recommend not skimping on these purchases. Yeah, you'll pay more for the organic whole food versions, but with the alternative chemicals mentioned, you're not absorbing them anyway, so, you might as well go for the good stuff. My opinion on supplementing, especially for peripheral neuropathy? Here you go:

- A great, organic, whole food based multivitamin/mineral listed above,
- A supplement that helps convert nitric oxide,
- Extra vitamin D3 (there will be some in the multi, but make sure you get at least a combined 2,000 I.U. per day)

In the next section, I'll go into more detail on these supplements and a few others and how to get them in your regular diet.

Nitric Oxide and the Nobel Prize

This molecule is formed naturally in our body and is known as a vasodilator, meaning that it helps to relax blood vessels, making them larger and easier for blood to pass through. Research into its function led to the 1998 Nobel Prize for discovering the role of nitric oxide as a cardiovascular signaling molecule. It's so critical to supporting the cardiovascular system by relaxing and dilating the arteries, I recommend it for nearly all of my neuropathy patients. Better circulation equals healthier tissues like nerves.

Now, you can't just buy Nitric Oxide, as it's formed inside of the arteries, but certain amino acids like L-Arginine, L-Citrulline and other vitamins like Vitamin D3 work synergistically to increase the natural production of nitric oxide.

Vitamin D helps our bodies in the absorption of calcium. Vitamin D also increases bone density and helps prevent bone fractures. Additionally, this vitamin helps regulate the immune system and protects against some types of cancer. Deficiency of Vitamin D has been linked to cancer, diabetes, osteoporosis, rheumatoid arthritis, inflammatory bowel disease, multiple sclerosis and autism. So, it's a pretty important vitamin, wouldn't you say? That's the main reason why I recommend supplementing it every day unless your doctor runs a blood test and determines that your levels are optimum (only likely if you often work and/or play outside).

Humans can synthesize their own vitamin D – all it takes is a bunch of regular sunshine. People in warm climates who often work or play in the sun rarely have vitamin D deficiencies. It's our neighbors to the north and those of us who are indoors most of the day who suffer. Couple this with bundling up in the colder seasons, the fear mongering skin cancer-phobes who recommend bathing in sunscreen 24/7, 365, and we create the perfect storm to have a whole nation who is woefully deficient in this very important vitamin (estimated at 70-85% of us). It's a very cheap vitamin to buy and I've even tested those sold at CVS and Walmart and found them to be good enough. How much? Depends on a lot of factors, but as a starting point, I encourage all of my patients over 12 to supplement with at least 2,000 IU (International Units) per day.

Vitamin B12

There's a sheath that surrounds our nerves made of a substance called myelin. It's kind of like the insulation that covers the wires in our homes. It's necessary to help the nerves work correctly and, when it is damaged or missing, neuropathy can ensue. Vitamin B12, which we must get from our diet, is necessary for the creation and preservation of this sheath. Too little B12 and you've got peripheral neuropathy (and other problems too). It is estimated that between 10% and 25% of the people over 80 years of age may have a B12 deficiency, so I'd recommend getting your levels checked. It's a simple blood test your doc can run. Not that you'd want to get it, but here is a list of great ways to acquire Vitamin B12 deficiency.

- alcoholism
- vegan diets
- certain autoimmune diseases
- pernicious or unexplained anemia
- pancreatic diseases
- ileal resection
- Irritable Bowel Syndrome or Crohn's Disease
- HIV infection
- Gastritis
- gastric or small intestine surgeries
- malabsorption syndromes
- multiple sclerosis
- histamine 2 receptor antagonists or proton pump inhibitors (medications)
- other OTC and prescription medications

Here are your best sources of B12

- red meat
- dairy products
- fish
- poultry and eggs
- A great, organic, whole food based multivitamin/mineral
- B12 injections are sometimes necessary

What Are Free Radicals?

Thomas Jefferson, Benjamin Franklin, Thomas Paine, and John Hancock were all radicals who wanted freedom for our country, but that's not the "free radicals" we're talking about in this section. In the human body, free radicals are formed when an electron in an atom becomes unpaired and searches for another electron to pair with. It may sound like an insignificant event, but this search for another unpaired atom causes damage to our cells and a chain reaction creating more free radicals.

Daily life exposes us to free radicals all the time, from the foods we eat to the air we breathe. Free radicals cause illness like peripheral neuropathy and contribute to the aging process. They have a negative impact on how we look and feel. Free radicals occur in everyday life but are made worse by:

- eating a diet full of processed foods and produce treated with chemicals
- smoking
- using drugs (prescription and over the counter)
- failure to deal correctly with stress
- excessive sun exposure
- pollution

Free radical damage can lead to:

- cancer
- heart disease
- diabetes
- arthritis
- autoimmune diseases
- peripheral neuropathy

One thing we can do to fight free radicals is to get more antioxidants in our diets. Antioxidants are vitamins, minerals, and other nutrients that protect the body and fight off free radicals. They give free radicals an electron to pair with before the stray electrons can damage our cells. Some examples of antioxidants are beta-carotene, Vitamin C, and Vitamin E. These vitamins help strengthen the immune system, too. Plus, they're readily available in many plant-based foods which we should consume more of anyway!

I will give examples of how to get more antioxidants into your system below but if you just follow the diet recommendations I laid out above, and vary your food intake (especially your fruits and veggies), you won't have to get a degree in nutrition science or memorize this list. But, for those of you who are interested in the topic, here is the list.

Beta-Carotene

Beta-Carotene is one of a group of red, orange, and yellow pigments called carotenoids. Beta-Carotene and other carotenoids provide approximately 50% of the

Vitamin A needed in our daily diet.[23] It's a powerful antioxidant that also helps protect the cells and boost the immune system. Sources of this vital nutrient include:

- carrots
- pumpkins
- sweet potatoes
- spinach
- collards
- kale
- turnip greens
- beet greens
- winter squash
- cabbage

If you would rather get your vitamin A straight-up instead of through the beta-carotene conversion, eat more:

- beef
- broccoli
- cantaloupe
- apricots
- liver
- whole eggs

---

[23] MedlinePlus (June 7, 2012). U.S. National Library of Medicine. Medline Plus Trusted Health Information for You. Beta-carotene. Retrieved from www.nlm.nih.gov/medlineplus/druginfo/natural/999.html.

Vitamin C

Vitamin C is another antioxidant that strengthens the immune system. It's vital to the growth and repair of skin, blood vessels, ligaments, and tendons. It is also involved with healing wounds and forming scar tissue. Plus, Vitamin C is important for the formation of collagen, which holds your body's cells together. And, it plays a significant role in maintaining oral and eye health.

Many fruits are excellent sources of vitamin C, including:

- cantaloupe
- orange
- citrus fruits
- kiwi
- mango
- guava
- papaya
- pineapple
- berries
- watermelon

You can get vitamin C from vegetables too, like cruciferous veggies (broccoli, cauliflower, and Brussels sprouts), peppers, leafy greens, potatoes, tomatoes, and squash.

Vitamin E

The third antioxidant we're concerned about is Vitamin E. This nutrient helps widen blood vessels and keeps blood from clotting inside them. Foods that are high in Vitamin E will also protect your skin from ultraviolet light, which is one of the leading causes of free radical formation in the body.

Excellent sources of vitamin E include:

- spinach
- chard
- turnip greens
- mustard greens
- cayenne pepper
- asparagus
- bell peppers
- eggs
- nuts and seeds
- meats
- olive oil
- whole grains

The next few (Magnesium, Calcium and Iron) are really minerals, but they play an essential part to many antioxidant reactions as well as many crucial body functions.

Magnesium is not only an essential mineral, but is responsible for over 300 healthy body functions. It also is the most deficient mineral in the Standard American Diet because it can be challenging to meet the daily requirements just from food. Less than 30% of U.S. adults consume the Recommended Daily Allowance of magnesium and nearly 20% of us get only half of the magnesium we need daily to remain healthy.[24]

To make sure you get enough magnesium in your diet, eat plenty of vegetables, nuts, seeds, dark chocolate, and seafood.

Calcium is the most abundant mineral in your body. It is responsible for strong teeth and bones, as well as proper function of blood vessels, nerve communication, and muscles. Many Americans suffer from a deficiency in calcium. We lose calcium each day through our skin, nails, hair, sweat, and waste.

To make sure you get enough calcium in your diet, make sure you consume:

- spinach
- broccoli
- kale
- Chinese cabbage
- salmon
- (and not dairy)

---

[24] LL Magnetic Clay Inc. (1996-2010). Ancient Minerals: Need More Magnesium? 10 Signs to Watch For. Retrieved from: www.ancient-minerals.com/magnesium-deficiency/need-more/.

Iron is important for the production of hemoglobin (found in red blood cells) and myoglobin (found in muscles). These proteins carry and store oxygen throughout the body. When you don't have enough iron in your body, you feel tired, weak, and unable to focus. Few people ever have too much iron in the body, but this rare condition is toxic.

Excellent sources of iron include:
- red meat
- liver
- egg yolks
- leafy green veggies
- dried fruits
- shellfish
- beans
- lentils
- artichokes

Pairing iron-rich foods with Vitamin C-rich foods will help your body absorb the iron better.[25]

It's hard to pare the whole topic of nutrition down into a single chapter, but, for peripheral neuropathy, I've listed out the most important issues. Basically, eat a superb, clean diet and take a few supplements to fill in the gaps. Oh, and drink a lot of water.

---

[25]WebMD. (2005–2012). Weight Loss & Diet Plans. Top 10 Iron-Rich Foods. Retrieved from: www.webmd.com/diet/features/top-10-iron-rich-foods.

Chapter 7

Low Level Light Therapy

Case Study

"I called in because I was having problems with severe headaches, dizziness, vertigo, nausea, acid reflux, fatigue and I'm only 31 years old! I had gone to a couple of doctors and they prescribed medications, and they weren't doing anything. It's sad to hear from a doctor that you are gonna have to learn to live with it and to just kind of give up.

After Dr. Prax's neuropathy program everything is so much better. My acid reflux has gotten completely better, I haven't had a headache in, I don't know how long, I've lost about 13 pounds and 2 inches off my belly. I believe that the dizziness/vertigo and nausea were all side effects of the medications and since I no longer take those, all of those symptoms are gone too.

I'm going to the fair tomorrow. That's something that last year at this time I never would have imagined doing. Now I don't even think twice about doing things like going out with my husband, cleaning the house or going to the park and walking my dog...I mean, my body's just - ABLE. This may seem like simple things but for

me, it's my life...I've got it back. It's just wonderful. I'm living again." Ana M.

Creating the Most Optimal Circulation

Remember the analogy I discussed in Chapter 5? The one about the houseplants that were in serious trouble after an extended vacation. We examined the survival instinct, known as "innate intelligence," which all living organisms possess. The bottom line was this: you can best help the plant by giving it what it needs, getting out of the way and allowing nature to take over. Then it had a pretty good chance to heal itself, right? The same thing is true for other organisms like humans, and their wilting nerves called neuropathy. We just need to give that body what it needs. One of the most important things a body needs to reverse neuropathy is a great blood flow to the damaged area. If there is poor circulation to your feet or hands then there's no way that the nerves in that region will be able to survive, let alone heal. Many of the following primary conditions cause poor circulation, which can lead to peripheral neuropathy:

- diabetes
- peripheral vascular disease (aka peripheral artery disease)
- atherosclerosis
- varicose veins
- obesity
- Raynaud's syndrome

If you are not getting adequate blood flow to those nerves then they are not receiving the nutrients they need to function. Not enough nutrients like glucose and oxygen? Nerves die. And that is called neuropathy. Nerves that are dying off send signals to the brain of pain, burning and tingling. In some cases, numbness ensues – no sensory signals are getting to the brain and it can't feel anything. Now, if the brain can't detect its own feet, it would make it hard for you to balance, right?

In addition to supplements that were mentioned in Chapter 6, Low Level Light Therapy (LLLT, aka Infrared Light Therapy) stimulates that oh-so-important Nitric Oxide. Remember that molecule? That is the one that relaxes (or dilates) the arteries, stimulates capillary growth and, therefore increases blood flow.

The Powerhouse of the Cell

At our most basic level, there is the human cell, and within that cell, there are little tiny organelles that have different jobs. The one we'll focus on here is called the mitochondria. It's known as the "powerhouse" of the cell. Its job is to make energy so that we can do stuff. This energy is called Adenosine Triphosphate, aka ATP. ATP is the fuel that all human cells utilize. This next part is very important, so follow along. In order to make ATP, the mitochondria must have two main ingredients – glucose and oxygen, both of which are carried to cells through blood flow. Turns out, the mitochondria are very sensitive to light and particularly Infrared Light. The depth of sunlight penetration is from 2-10 mm. Infrared light (not visible to our eye) penetrates up to 100 mm (that's up to 4 inches) deep.

Stimulating the mitochondria increases its activity which increases the fuel needed to repair cells. It's a good thing! When we increase circulation with LLLT together with the nitric oxide boosting supplement, we are giving the mitochondria the ingredients it needs to make the fuel to heal those nerves.

Here are some other benefits of nitric oxide:
- anti-inflammatory
- aids in tissue regeneration
- pain reduction
- increases localized circulation
- lowers blood pressure
- reduces angina
- helps reverse erectile dysfunction (Viagra, Cialis, and Levitra work on nitric oxide pathways to increase blood flow to the penis and substantially improve erections)
- protection against dementia and other neurodegenerative disorders
- improves digestion
- improves insulin signaling
- improves bone remodeling
- better respiratory function

- improves ATP (energy) utilization

What Role Does LLLT Play in Treating Peripheral Neuropathy?

Because LLLT (Low Level Light Therapy) stimulates cellular regeneration, it plays a vital role in a complete treatment plan for peripheral neuropathy patients. LLLT helps damaged nerves and their surrounding blood vessels regrow, gradually improving sensation and function for the patient. There are currently no drugs on the market that can help the body heal itself in such a way. Plus, unlike virtually all medications, there are absolutely no side effects associated with LLLT. The area may feel warm or tingly during the treatment, but there are no other reported physical sensations from LLLT patients.

When a patient visits our office for treatment of peripheral neuropathy, we apply LLLT boots around the hands, feet, or both and let the machine deliver the treatment for a specified amount of time. Some of our moderate and severe cases and/or remote cases will receive both the supplement and the best LLLT unit to use at home. Patients can then receive treatments daily and sometimes twice daily.

Chapter 8

Electrotherapy

Case Study

When Sheree first came to us, she reported throbbing, aching pain and occasional sharp shooting pains and cramping in her legs and feet. She also had issues with swelling and lower back pain from a fall from years earlier.

Sheree was a very active person who was on her feet all the time and stated that she wasn't the type to just sit around, despite the pain. She complained that even when she wasn't on her feet, they still hurt 24/7. It was waking her up 3-4 times a night and she was taking Tylenol and Benadryl to attempt to sleep through it.

Six weeks after she started the program, Sheree reported that the program, "especially the Rebuilder®," was significantly helping. At that reevaluation, she reported a 45% improvement.

A few weeks later, on a weekend trip to New York City with her daughter, she went off the diet and stopped using the Rebuilder®. She reasoned that she was feeling so much better, and, with this new lease on life, she was going to have some fun! That following Monday she lamented that she was "all the way back to square one. Everything has come back."

Well, per my suggestion she "got back in the saddle," put herself back on the diet and resumed her therapies. Weeks later she had this to say. "When I first started here, I was in extreme pain...I was bottomed out. I couldn't get any worse. Doing your program has made a huge difference in my life. I know I'm only going to continue to get better. I have lost over 20 pounds and I feel so much better. I am sleeping all the way through the night without any medications now. I feel 10 times better, in my back, my feet and in every way.

Sheree serves as a great example of the importance of sticking to the program, and, even if you "fall off the horse," you just need to climb back up there and take it one step at a time.

Right off the bat, let's get one thing out of the way: this is nothing like the practice of electroshock therapy that was used in asylums decades ago. On the other hand, it's more exciting than the electrolysis procedure that can get rid of unwanted body hair.

With few exceptions, I prescribe a tool that actually stimulates growth in the nerves that are dying off from peripheral neuropathy. I've tried many similar tools, but time and again, I keep coming back to the ReBuilder®.

It is an FDA-approved device that was designed specifically to treat the pain, burning, numbness, and tingling associated with peripheral neuropathy. In fact, The Cancer Treatment Centers of America®, Johns Hopkins, Harvard Medical School, the Cleveland Clinic, Memorial Sloan Kettering Cancer Centers, and others use the ReBuilder® to alleviate their patients' chemotherapy-induced neuropathy. We've been using it effectively since 2010, and it's worked very well for us.

What does the ReBuilder® do?

When first turned on, your ReBuilder® evaluates your body's electrical state and it then sets itself for your safety. It can tell the difference between a 100 lb person and a 300 lb athlete. Thus, it is self-limiting.

It then sends a healthy nerve signal from foot to foot (or hand to hand) and then goes quiet to "listen" to the self-generated response to that signal that the body sends up to your brain. It copies and evaluates that (dysfunctional) signal and compares it to a proper signal and creates a custom compensating signal, like a pacemaker does for your heart signal. It then sends this signal 7.83 times per second to gently coax your nerves to relearn how to send a healthy signal that can reach the brain.

This is a very slow signal that relaxes the brain and encourages it to release endorphins that travel throughout your body via your blood stream to help you relax, reduce pain in other parts of your body, and helps you get to sleep at night. Nerve impulses travel in excess of 240 miles per hour, so there is a relatively large resting phase between each ReBuilder® signal to enable your nerves to absorb oxygen and other nutrients.

The ReBuilder® evaluates your dysfunctional nerves and creates a compensating signal (like a Bose noise-canceling headphone) 7.83 times per second and your nerves will begin to heal during the 30-minute treatment.

The ReBuilder® also stimulates your nearby calf muscles to stimulate the venous muscle pump to increase local blood flow while it strengthens those muscles to avoid disuse muscle atrophy. This action has a second benefit, as the increased blood flow (to the entire lower half of your body when treating the feet) causes a beneficial "shear stress" resulting from the increased velocity inside your veins and this action releases vast amounts of nitric oxide, which opens the capillaries to increase blood flow and stimulate angiogenesis (the development of new blood vessels). When used together with the Low Level Lights I discussed in the previous chapter, even better results can be attained.

When used simultaneously with the warm water foot bath, the warm water expands the blood vessels in your feet and ankles (vasodilatation) to allow more blood to reach your nerves and skin. This is especially beneficial for people suffering from diabetes. The ReBuilder® has a built-in timer that turns itself off after the relaxing 30-minute treatment.

What Are the Benefits of ReBuilder® Treatment?

Daily, thirty-minute ReBuilder® treatments in your home may significantly reduce the amount of pain medications needed to deal with an acute pain syndrome. This is especially desirable considering all drugs have side effects and many of them are symptoms of neuropathy. The fewer drugs you are on, the fewer the side effects – a great thing!

ReBuilder® also increases blood flow, strengthens muscles, and improves the transmission of signals within the nervous system, and when patients experience less pain at night, they tend to get a better night's sleep. This allows them to function better during the daytime and promotes cellular repair and regeneration during their restful hours.

The effects of this treatment method are cumulative, meaning that the longer you continue to use it, the better the results you will see. In both moderate and severe cases I'll recommend a home unit so that my patients can use it daily. I have some very complex cases that'll actually use it 2 or 3 times daily. As they progress through more and more treatments, their condition improves and the need for electrotherapy is reduced.

Whether your peripheral neuropathy is a side effect of statin drugs, chemotherapy treatment, diabetes, or any other of the known 100+ causes, ReBuilder® can help restore function and sensation to your peripheral nervous system.

Please keep in mind that my approach is a well rounded one, designed to take care of as many "straws on the camel's back" as possible. I've consulted with many patients who came to me frustrated that they tried the Rebuilder® (and other products available online) only to discover that it didn't help at all. The ReBuilder® is incredible but it is only one piece in the puzzle in our innovative program. I strongly believe that a more complete approach to neuropathy is a smarter plan of action. That's why we prescribe electrotherapy, low level light therapy, Brain-Based Therapy, nutrition, and vibration therapy to our patients who are struggling to get their pain under control and live an active life like they desire.

Chapter 9

Brain-Based Therapy

Case Study

Here's a case where Sherlock Holmes could have been helpful. Susan, a relatively healthy, young (48 year old) female who exercised regularly and watched her diet carefully, presented to my office with terrible symptoms of peripheral neuropathy (severe numbness and pain at the same time).

In addition, she experienced frequent severe migraine headaches, low back pain, neck pain, irritable bowel syndrome, GERD and pernicious anemia. She admitted to smoking 1/2 a pack a day and rarely drank alcohol.

This poor soul was super motivated to get well. The doctors had her on five different medications for her various symptoms and she was injecting herself daily with B12 just HOPING for ANY relief. She had been to more than a handful of doctors, none of whom were able to figure it out. They called it "idiopathic neuropathy," and I agreed. I couldn't find a cause for it either, but she definitely had neuropathy. Her Toronto Scoring Index indicated a 55% loss of the sensory nerves in her feet.

Even though I could not find a cause, we decided to start her on our all-natural neuropathy protocols. She followed them all to a "T."She completely changed her diet, went cold turkey on the smoking, stopped drinking and used the at-home therapies exactly as directed. Within a month her IBS and GERD had improved significantly, she had lost 13 pounds, the sinus pain was gone and her back pain was better – but the foot pain was still there... it hadn't budged at all.

At this point, it was time to pull out my Sherlock Holmes hat and go to work. Upon further questioning, I found out that around 3 years previously, the room that she had been working in was remodeled. "Why?" I asked (remodels can leave behind nasty chemicals from things like paint, carpets, and glues). Turns out there had been a slow water leak from the AC unit and, as a result, the wooden floor was buckling.

This was right next to where Susan was sitting 8 hours a day. I wanted her employer to pull a few of the floorboards and sheetrock to see if there was any mold, but she was really reticent to ask her boss to go through all that trouble.
She finally was able to get the maintenance guy to inspect by lifting up the heater vent. When he reported "nothing," I was still skeptical. It really needed a thorough investigation but what if they

pulled floorboards and sheetrock and it came back clear? It was a lot to ask, but Susan's health and life depended on it.

There was another way, I explained to her. We could run a blood test which is what we ended up doing. Guess what? It came back positive for mold. We couldn't identify what strand of mold or even it where it came from but her body was definitely reacting to it. Immediately she relocated to another space in the office and she was referred to a natural mold specialist where she was put on a detox program. I learned a valuable lesson in this case.

Although I was not the one to finally rid her of her neuropathy, I was the one who was able to find the underlying cause of her neuropathy. Not one of her medications would EVER get rid of the mold toxicity that she was breathing in, day in and day out. SHE needed to be removed from the source and then the mold needed to be removed from her body.

Moral of the story? SOMEBODY MUST find the underlying cause of the neuropathy or it'll NEVER be solved. Case closed.

Brain-Based Therapy (BBT) is an amazingly powerful, all-natural healing technique used to restore people to their optimum state of health.

How does the brain work?

Your brain controls and coordinates all functions of the body. Most people have learned that the left side of the brain controls the right side of the body. Additionally, the right side of the body feeds sensory information to the left side of your brain and, of course, the left side of the body feeds sensory information to the right side of the brain. Here's where it gets a little confusing. When folks refer to the "brain," they are usually talking about the larger parts called the Cerebrum.

Well, there are other parts too and, for this book, we only need to know about two of those parts. We must talk about the Cerebellum. The Cerebellum controls the SAME side of the body – it doesn't cross to the other side. Also, it talks to the Cerebrum, but, confusingly, it is "wired" to the OPPOSITE side of the Cerebrum. When functioning normally, the Cerebellum, which is located in the lower part of your cranium, sends messages, or "fires," to the opposite side brain, which, in turn, "fires" to the brainstem (mesencephalon, pons, and medulla). This is called the "Brain Loop" and it looks like this:

Normal Brain Function

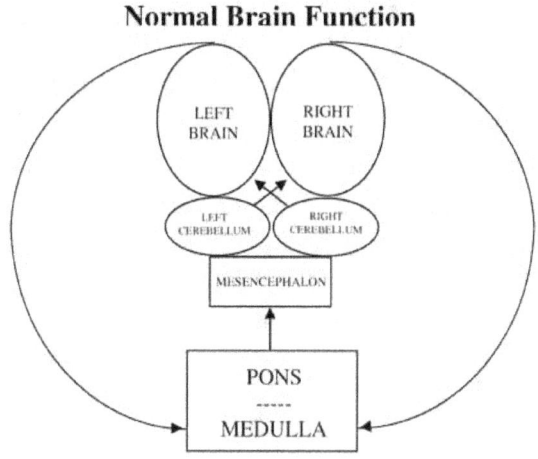

What does all this mean? You don't need to be a neuroscientist or really even need to understand exactly how the Brain Loop works, but you do need to know this: *your health, well-being, physical vitality, mental clarity, and emotional stability are all directly correlated with proper brain function – the "brain loop."*

What can go wrong?

Well, in a word, Stress…physical, chemical, and emotional stress will adversely affect this "brain loop." Stress is not necessarily a bad thing, however, it is the constant, pervasive, never-ending stress of our culture that is so detrimental. Too much stress, for too long will create an improper cascade of events that basically spins out of control, leading to neurological, hormonal, and other negative outcomes.

One example of this would be "cerebellar dysfunction." If one side of the cerebellum is not receiving the proper nerve input from the body, it cannot send sufficient nerve input to the opposite side frontal lobe, which, in turn, can't send enough input to the lower brainstem to keep the mesencephalon (midbrain) from over firing. It would look like this:

Abnormal Brain Function

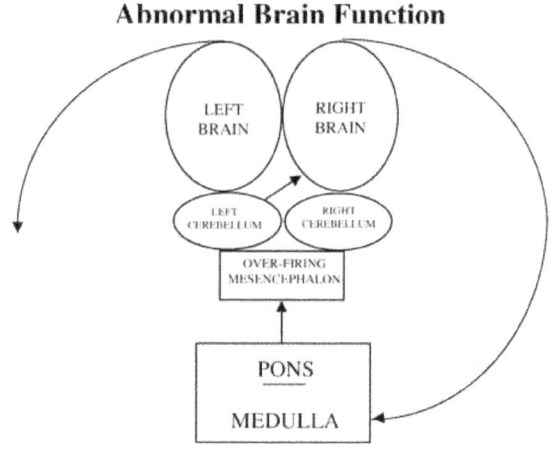

What's the deal with the mesencephalon?

The mesencephalon (a.k.a. midbrain) normally is inhibited by the brain. In other words, when the "brain loop" is intact, the mesencephalon is turned off (or on low). However, once stress interrupts the "brain loop," the mesencephalon is left unchecked. Basically, the brain gets stuck in a sympathetic (fight or flight) response, which is like a stuck accelerator in your car. Below are some of the symptoms of an over-firing mesencephalon.

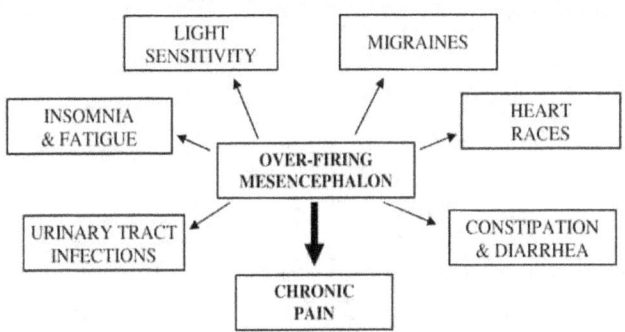

What about the Cerebellum?

As mentioned, another key part to the "brain loop" is the Cerebellum. This is the back, bottom part of your brain that controls your balance and coordination, spinal postural muscles, and helps control eye movements (and much, much more). When one side of your Cerebellum is not firing properly, it can lead to a host of common ailments.

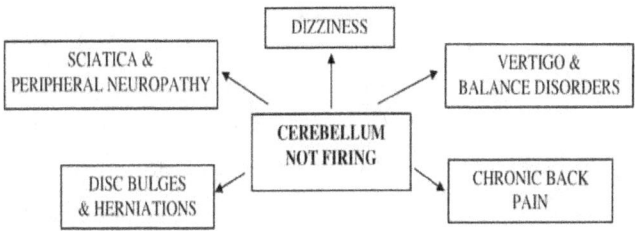

A misfiring Cerebellum will cause one side of the postural muscles to be tighter than the other side. This asymmetrical muscle tone will cause imbalances throughout the body. Often, individual vertebrae will lock up and be restricted in their normal movement.

Consequently, chronic back and/or neck pain, spinal degeneration (arthritis), disc herniation, and/or sciatica may develop. Also, once pathologies are ruled out, chronic dizziness and balance disorders are usually the result of cerebellar dysfunction.

How do you fix the brain?

Neuroplasticity: The ability of the brain to form and reorganize synaptic connections, especially in response to learning or experience or following injury.

Most of us learned in biology 101 that "once a nerve or brain tissue has been damaged, it cannot be regenerated." Well, that's just not true. The word for this is "neuroplasticity" and, basically, it means that a damaged nerve CAN be regenerated.

Think about what would happen if you broke your arm and had to have it in a cast for six months. What would happen? Your muscles (and bones) would atrophy, right? They'd become smaller and weaker. Well, with the correct exercises, over time, you could get them to grow back. Turns out the same exact thing can happen with damaged nerves – you just need to know how to exercise, and in turn, stimulate the nerves correctly.

Now, let's go a little deeper into the neurology of peripheral neuropathy. There are receptors, specialized nerve endings, that feel things from the environment such as hot, cold, pressure, vibration, pain and more that are located throughout the body. By definition, *sensory neurons* are nerve cells within the nervous system responsible for converting external stimuli from the organism's environment into electrical impulses.

The electrical impulses are carried over wires, which we call nerves, from the receptor all the way up to the brain, where they are interpreted as a sensation. If we are looking at the foot, for example, the first nerve to carry the impulse from the receptor is called the peripheral nerve and it travels all the way up your leg to the spinal cord in the lower back where the first connection is made. Some of these second nerves cross to the other side of the spinal cord right there and some of them cross over higher up in the brain stem.

Either way, they all cross to the other side of the brain and eventually end up in the "Parietal Lobe" in the brain. This lobe is otherwise known as the "sensory cortex," that area of the brain that is responsible for interpreting these electrical impulses. Our brain decodes those impulses as pain, vibration, hot, cold, etc. Pretty neat, huh?

The Key to Neuropathy

So, with that very brief description of the amazing nervous system, here's the takeaway. **Any** of the aforementioned areas could be damaged. More often than not, more than one will be damaged. What if your practitioner is only taking care of the receptors, but the peripheral nerve itself is damaged. Don't forget about the spinal cord, brain stem, cerebellum and even the brain itself. Someone must check the entire pathway, from receptors in the feet and hands all the way up to the brain itself. It's akin to a hose that is not allowing water to run through it. Someone must check the entire length of the hose for kinks, not just at either end.

The challenge of figuring out peripheral neuropathy

There are over 100 known causes of peripheral neuropathy. There are so many different things that can go wrong that figuring out the cause of it can be quite a challenge. It could be actual damage at the receptor, damage at the peripheral nerve that carries the information from the receptor, damage at the spinal cord, brainstem or even the brain itself. In reality, most cases have damage at more than one of these nerve pathways.

The number one cause of peripheral neuropathy is related to diabetes or blood sugar regulation issues. If that's the only problem, then getting the blood glucose regulation under control is paramount to correcting the underlying nerve damage. If the cause is chemically related, such as chemotherapy, Agent Orange, antibiotic or some other prescription medication, then that would require a separate strategy.

What if, in addition to anything listed above, the patient also has arthritis of the lower back; maybe some scoliosis, or even a bulging disk? Those additional "straws on the camel's back" would need to be considered as well. What if your neuropathy is caused by your cholesterol-lowering statin medication? Well, if that's the case, then looking at the liver is a key component. The liver is what is creating the cholesterol, which is the reason why your doctor is prescribing the medication in the first place. Most of these problems can be resolved or greatly affected by dietary and exercise modifications.

Medical doctors are usually pretty good at diagnosing peripheral neuropathy and they have a number of different diagnostic tools at their disposal. MRI, EMG, CT scans and blood labs are some of the tools which can help them identify exactly where the problem is and how bad it is. But what then? So your doctor or neurologist gives you the results of the studies and tells you, "You have moderate to severe neuropathy in your lower extremities."

Most of the time, my patients want to say to the doctor, "Gee doc, I could have told you that!" The real question they should be asking, though, is, "What can we do about this neuropathy?" The medical answer is almost always "more medication". However, for most neuropathy causes, you will never be able to medicate this problem away.

Anyway, what's most important to understand for correcting peripheral neuropathy? First, and foremost, you must know what the cause is. We must know what it is that is failing so that we can support that system of the body. Number two, we need to set realistic expectations. Some cases of neuropathy will never heal up 100%, and some cases may not heal at all – it's just too far gone. For those cases which I know I can help, we start with a strategy that simply works to eliminate the offending activity. If it's too much blood sugar, then diet must be addressed.

A thorough *functional* neurological examination will reveal which aspect of your brain is not firing properly. Since one side of the body is controlled by the opposite side of the brain (example: right brain controls the left side of the body), most treatments are given on one side of the body to stimulate the opposite hemisphere of the brain.

A safe, gentle, hands-on, dynamic integration process is used to reboot, reconnect and restore proper brain function. Traditional chiropractic instruments and/or adjustments are also used, but they are used in a very precise manner…to stimulate function in the affected part of the brain.

In addition, visual, auditory, and olfactory stimulation, heat, eye movements, eye exercises, and other modalities may be used to increase brain firing.

What Health Problems Can BBT Help With?

Please understand that BBT is not a specific treatment for any disease, illness or disorder. We do not try to cure anything. Our expertise lies in naturally and holistically rewiring your brain and then getting out of the way so your body can heal. However, once the "brain loop" is restored and any brain imbalances are minimized...amazing things can happen. The following is a list of health conditions people have shown significant improvement with:

- balance disorders
- arm/shoulder pain
- low back pain/sciatica
- bulging/herniated discs
- carpal tunnel syndrome
- dizziness
- dystonia
- early Alzheimer's symptoms
- Fibromyalgia
- RLS (restless leg syndrome)
- headaches
- migraines
- insomnia
- hip/knee/feet pain
- tremor disorders
- MS symptoms
- neck pain
- numbness
- spinal stenosis
- low immunity

Who Discovered BBT?

Brain-Based Therapy is a clinical, functional neurological protocol developed by Dr. Fred Carrick, the country's leading chiropractic neurologist and chiropractic's only neurological fellow. The Carrick

Institute offers classes internationally and helps patients around the world with severe neurological disorders.

In addition, Dr. Andy Barlow, a board certified chiropractic neurologist, out of Tupelo, MS, and CEO of the American Functional Neurology Institute (AFNI), has developed a BBT/Neurological program for chiropractors in the United States who wish to pursue this post graduate training. I became certified in 2013 and continue to update my certification annually.

We have been working closely with Dr. Barlow and the AFNI to ensure that the patients at our office can benefit from this amazing approach to overall health.

Chapter 10

Vibration Therapy

Case Study

My doctor had suggested I call Dr. Prax because I was having back pain, leg pain and foot pain. Driving and standing was especially painful and standing all day is what I do for a living! I saw Dr. Prax and his whole treatment was completely different from anything I'd seen. I noticed an improvement after the first session. Of all the different therapies he uses, the vibration platform is one of my favorites. The energy that I feel from it goes up from the feet to the legs and to my back. It's wonderful.

When you walk so stiff and you're hurting all the time and you're popping whatever pills you can get just to get through the day, you need to look for another way. Thanks to my medical doctor for sending me here. I swear by Dr. Prax's program. It's just totally different. Sage G.

Healthcare providers, physical therapists, occupational therapists, chiropractors, and personal trainers use whole body vibration therapy (WBVT), for a surprisingly wide range of purposes. Specifically, vibration therapy is great for:

- increasing muscle endurance, coordination, and strength
- better circulation of lymph fluid and blood for better healing, energy, and overall health
- improving nerve activity
- boosting bone density and fighting off osteoporosis

Here's an unbelievable story about WBVT and my mother-in-law. At 75, she found her bone density levels to be quite severe. Unfortunately, she was following her mother's lead with this debilitating condition. Broken bones, back and hip pain, stooped posture, and decreasing height are the most common symptoms of it and she did not want anything to do with any of those.

Her integrative, out-of-the-box thinking medical doctor (Dr. Zach Bush), recommended that she purchase a whole body vibration therapy unit and that she use it every day for a minimum of 10 minutes.

Religiously, she followed the recommendation for a year and her bone density was rechecked. Dr. Bush was blown away at how little bone loss occurred in all her body and how, in some areas, there was actually bone GROWTH! This is astonishing because in western medicine, no one gets better with osteoporosis. Even the medications for it like Fosamax have shown little evidence of actually helping with bone strengthening;

some research shows that these drugs can INCREASE the risk of fracture. Anyway, suffice it to say I find it to be very helpful for bone density.

And, there's more: for my patients with peripheral neuropathy, vibration therapy reduces their pain, increases circulation, improves strength and flexibility, and increases energy, mobility, and balance. Of course, these results are achieved without drugs or invasive surgery.

A recent study showed that patients with Diabetic Peripheral Neuropathy (DPN) specifically have much to gain from vibration therapy. Study participants were observed to determine how effective whole body vibration therapy really is in treating pain associated with DPN. The study's participants received three whole body vibration treatments per week for a month. Each session consisted of four rounds of three minutes of vibration.

The study's results demonstrated significant pain reduction overall, and no side effects were observed during the study.[26] With less pain and better sensation, patients are likely to see far fewer serious injuries and infections due to increased sensation and better coordination.

---

[26] "Why Use VibePlate for Vibration Therapy, Vibration Training, & Vibration Exercise." N.p., n.d. Web. 26 July 2015. <http://www.vibeplate.net/why-vibeplate>.

How Does WBVT Work?

Vibration therapy devices come in a range of forms. In our office, we have vibrating foot platforms that treat just peripheral neuropathy of the feet. We also use hand-held devices to target very specific areas of the body and fully customize the length and duration of treatment. The advantage with these is that they are very cheap. (My current favorite is the "HoMedics Percussion Action Handheld Massager with Heat." It can be found online for under $40).

We also have the standing vibration platform which is what is called Whole Body Vibration Therapy. If they can tolerate it, we have our neuropathy patients stand on the platform for a full-body treatment. Either way, the high frequency vibration is an effective and safe treatment for the area(s) of the body affected by neuropathy.

Vibration therapy stimulates a patient's muscles to rapidly contract. Frequent tightening of a muscle will build and strengthen the muscle tissue, even when it's performed for small bits of time. As the muscle builds, its need for blood also grows. This is what stimulates blood vessels to grow and keep fueling the muscles with the nutrients they need during and after vibration therapy.

It's important to note that while traditional exercise is difficult and often uncomfortable for many patients dealing with chronic pain, vibration therapy cuts these complications out of the equation. When people have reduced sensation in their feet and hands, it can be downright dangerous to pick up free weights or hop onto a treadmill, but vibration therapy allows the patient to stand or even sit throughout the "workout," as muscles are being strengthened the entire time.

When the muscles are pushed and exerted in specific ways, they in turn stimulate the nerves connected to them and can, therefore, regrow their pathways and even repair or rebuild the damaged nerves.

An added bonus of vibration therapy is that it stimulates the osteoblasts. Osteoblasts are cells that make it possible for bones to grow stronger by creating new bone cells. Did you catch that? Vibration therapy has been proven to stimulate bone growth.

Neurologically, stimulating the vibration nerve receptors, called Pacinian corpuscles, causes an inhibition of pain nerves. Stimulating those vibration pathways regularly, over a long period of time (at least a month) will create stronger vibration signals, more vibration nerves and more receptive vibration receptors. Bottom line? Vibration therapy reduces pain signals that fire up to the brain. This is a good thing for neuropathy, right?

All of these facts combined means that vibration therapy patients will regain sensation, strength, and stamina and reduce pain signals.. Over time, the little things in life that used to be exhausting will become far easier. Eventually, patients get back to more normal routines and introduce regular moderate exercise to their daily calendars. It is truly an eye-opening experience to lose full use of parts of your body, and then gain it back again. Your priorities and your perspective will never be the same.

Is There Anybody Who Should NOT Experience WBVT?

Certain patients should not participate in vibration therapy, including patients with epilepsy, severe vertigo, or a detached retina. Also, if you are pregnant, vibration therapy is probably not safe for you.

The Keys to Neuropathy Reversal

To effectively treat chronic conditions, like peripheral neuropathy, we must approach it using several different modalities. That's why we never treat a neuropathy patient with just vibration therapy. Our neuropathy patients commonly experience vibration therapy, low-level light therapy, soft tissue treatments, electrical stimulation, spinal decompression and Brain-Based Therapy during their visits. We go at these conditions with everything we've got because patient comfort, health, and satisfaction are paramount. We know that this multi-pronged approach is the best way to get people off painkillers and back on their feet. Having said that, if you can afford a standing vibration platform, GET IT! At minimum purchase a hand held vibration massager. Subscribe to my YouTube channel (Dr. Brian Prax) and watch my videos on how to use these devices. It's free to subscribe.

Chapter 11

Soft Tissue Therapies

Case Study

Our patient Joseph M. gave his testimonial after going through our Knee Pain and Lower Back Pain and Sciatica program. According to him, his lower back pain is "100% BETTER and knee pain is 99% BETTER. My back pain when gardening was unbearable and my favorite hobby, scuba diving was getting harder and harder. After the first session it was at least 80% better. With the Trigenics, the pressure, the manipulation you do, and your [Arthrostim] I'm able to garden again. It's wonderful."

Trigenics® – a Miracle Technique

In all the 20 plus years I've been a chiropractor, I have never seen anything so powerful as the technique called Trigenics® and we frequently turn to it in our neuropathy program. From the website, www.trigenics.com:

> Trigenics® is an advanced neurological muscle assessment, treatment and training system which instantly reprograms the way the brain communicates with the body to immediately

relieve pain, amplify strength and movement and augment muscular performance.

The complex multimodal procedures in Trigenics® simultaneously combine three exercise and treatment protocols for a much greater therapeutic and training enhancement effect than ever before thought possible.

I have seen so many jaw-dropping results from this technique and it continually blows my mind! It is most commonly used with our knee pain program, yet we also employ it for neuropathy when needed. The definition above lays it all out correctly, and I like to explain it like this: it is similar to a combination of deep tissue massage and physical exercise at the same time.

The practitioner performs certain holds on specific muscles in very well-defined positions while the patient is making specific movements of the limbs. Instantaneous improvements are noticed by the patients almost every time. The technique works exceptionally well when there are limited ranges of motion, tight or cramping muscles or even with painful muscle regions. It can be a technique which finds very tender spots to be sure, so we always walk a patient through it, explaining as we go.

For more interesting before and after videos you can go to www.trigenics.com or my own website, http://www.chroniccarecharlottesville.com/knee-pain/.

Often a patient reports feeling lighter, or tells us that the tightness has lifted. In the next chapter, I'll discuss another technique that'll really loosen things up.

Trigger Point Therapy

l find Trigger Point Therapy to be very helpful especially when performed in the back and shoulders. A "trigger point" is a tight area within muscle tissue that causes pain to radiate to other parts of the body. A trigger point in the back, for example, may produce referred pain in the legs or even the knees. I've had this myself and it can be, not only very bothersome and painful, but also very confusing, until it's rectified. With an Arthrostim, which uses gentle percussions, or manually with a thumb or finger, a Trigger point can be worked out eliminating the referred pain. Many massage therapists are trained in this technique.

Massage Therapy

Massage therapy has been around for ages, it feels tremendous and can really help with the symptoms of peripheral neuropathy. There are many different techniques and each therapist has his or her own specialties. Getting those knots and stiffnesses worked out can make the difference between a "doable day" and one filled with suffering. We have an amazing one in our office but if you are not close by, ask around to find a skilled massage therapist.

Stretching and Yoga

The practice of yoga dates back to the 5th or 6th Century and it originated in India. It was initially created as a group of physical, mental and spiritual practices, but many modern yoga studios, or even yoga instructors online use it as a great way to stretch your muscles, build strength, work on balance and meditate. It doesn't have to interfere with your own spiritual belief, just take from it what you want. Personally I find it to be extremely helpful and it feels fantastic. I ALWAYS feel better, even after just 10 minutes of yoga stretching. Nowadays there is so much that the internet can provide. Try googling "stretches for lower back pain" or for sciatica, or even for peripheral neuropathy. It's amazing how helpful these stretches can be. Give it a whirl...I think you'll like it too.

Chapter 12

Spinal Decompression Therapy

Case Study

At the young age of 83, I got to where I could hardly walk anymore and I was carrying too much weight. I was in excruciating pain most of the time, so I decided to do something about it.

When I first started coming in here for treatment it was for my feet and for my back and legs. I had considerable leg damage from a total of 8 back surgeries. I have rods in my back but I came in here with a lot of pain in my feet, legs <u>and</u> back. Since going through [Dr. Prax's neuropathy program], I'm able to work 6 hours a day now instead of 2. That's quite an improvement and it's a lot of fun to be able to get out and do things on my farm.

My number one thing is hunting and fishing, I live to hunt and fish. I like to make things in my workshop and I just love to get on my buggies and ride around the mountain, enjoy the outdoors. It was very limiting. I could not put my shoes on myself, I couldn't get my socks on and I was getting tired of people coming around to get my socks off or my shoes on. I can get my socks on

**now, I can get my shoes on and off, I can get my
clothes on and off, so my wife gets a break. Best of
all is that I'm looking forward to hunting season!**

Al B.

As previously mentioned, most neuropathy cases have
more than one cause. We use "the straws on a camel's
back" analogy. In other words, even though 30% of all
neuropathies come from diabetes, there's over 100
known causes and one of those, almost always seen, is
nerve compression. If the nerves that exit the lower
back and go down to the legs and feet or the nerves that
leave the neck and go down into the arms and hands
are being compressed, pain, tingling, numbness or other
symptoms ensue.

Compression in the spine involving the disc and the
nerves themselves can obviously cause pain at the spine,
but not always; that's what makes it so tricky. The
sources of pain can be directly from the disc, or the disc
putting pressure on the nerves themselves. Here are the
most common ways nerves in the spine can become
compressed:

- misalignment of the spine
- scoliosis or curvatures
- osteoarthritis
- disc degeneration
- disc herniation

- disc bulging
- inflammation
- infection
- tumors of the spine
- rheumatoid arthritis

It is very important to differentially diagnose the cause(s) of the compression and your practitioner will most likely do an X-ray, MRI or CT scan to see what's going on.

Surgeons perform an operation called "spinal decompression" where they go in and decompress the vertebra. It involves removing some of the bone or disc around the spinal cord or the nerves that exit the spine– it's quite invasive. In our office, we use a much gentler technique called Non-Surgical Spinal Decompression Therapy (SDT). It has been around in one form or another for decades and there have been a great deal of studies on the therapy.

What we do is lay a patient down on the table (face up or face down) put on a lap belt, and the machine does all the rest for us. It actually decompresses the vertebrae and the discs in between. Honestly, it feels so good some of our patients fall asleep on it. A few things can happen with SDT:

- reduces disc pressure
- enhances disc healing

- facilitates a pumping action to the discs which pumps in oxygen, protein and other substrates, and pumps out waste products like carbon dioxide
- inhibits leakage of disc material
- vacuum effect; pulls disc material that has protruded back into the disc

Here are some of the most common ailments that SDT can treat:

- herniated disc
- degenerative disc disease
- sciatica
- facet syndrome
- post-surgical patient
- peripheral neuropathy from compressed nerves

As with all therapies there are relative contraindications and here is the list:

- disc fragmentation
- calcification
- severe arthritis
- surgical spinal appliances
- osteoporosis
- pars defect
- spondylolisthesis
- paralysis

If you have one or more of the above "relative contraindications," that just means we need to be extra careful, not that you absolutely cannot have the therapy. I take it case by case, but almost always use the therapy, albeit, starting very slowly and gently.

The Difference between Spinal Decompression Therapy (SDT) and Traction

I get this question occasionally. "What do you think about traction or an inversion table?" My answer is quite simple. "Well, what do YOU think about it?" because most times the question is asked from a patient who owns or has tried an inversion table or traction device. If they answer that they **love** it, I'd say, "Well, sounds good to me – keep doing it." If they have never tried it, then I explain the difference, so here goes:

"Spinal Traction" is defined as a continuous pulling with the same amount of force. This can be accomplished with yoga or stretching utilizing the "forward fold" move where you basically bend over, placing your chest on your thighs and really concentrate on relaxing – this can feel really good. It can also be accomplished using an inversion table where you'd strap your ankles (or hook your knees) into a table while upright and then rotate it to the "inverted" position (hanging upside down).

That can also feel lovely, but in both cases, start out slowly because if you are not used to being upside down and having your blood rush up to your head, it can be a dizzying experience! For the inversion table, I also recommend starting with NO MORE than 30 seconds and working your way up to maybe a few minutes. Also, make sure to have someone with you to help upright you if needed. This therapy can help with muscle spasms and even disc pain but it doesn't shine as well as SDT in the research.

Here's what an Inversion Table looks like:

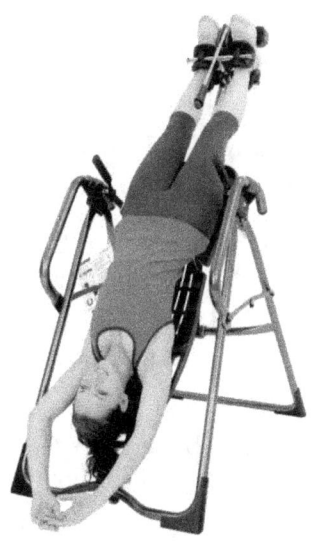

The difference with Spinal Decompression Therapy is with the application of forces. Whereas traction uses a continuous (often your body weight) force, SDT machines vary the forces. A patient lays either on their back or belly depending on the circumstance and is then hooked up to the device. For the lower back, a strap is wrapped around the pelvis and connected to the cable of the SDT machine. Next, an upper body strap is applied or, in some cases, an armpit bolster can be used – either one of these works to hold the upper body in place while the lower body is being pulled.

A computer is programmed considering a patient's height, weight, age, body type and other factors (osteoporosis, diabetes, and post-surgical to name a few). The machine always starts out with a very light force, usually 5 pounds, and pulls for around 30 seconds. It then takes much of the weight off, allowing for a resting period. This period is usually the same amount of time as the pulling time.

Next, a greater force, say 10 pounds is applied for 30 seconds, then rest. This continues in a pyramid fashion. In other words, the force goes up to a max, with resting in between pulls, and then it works its way back down to smaller forces. Here's what our SDT table looks like when used for lumbar (lower back) SDT.

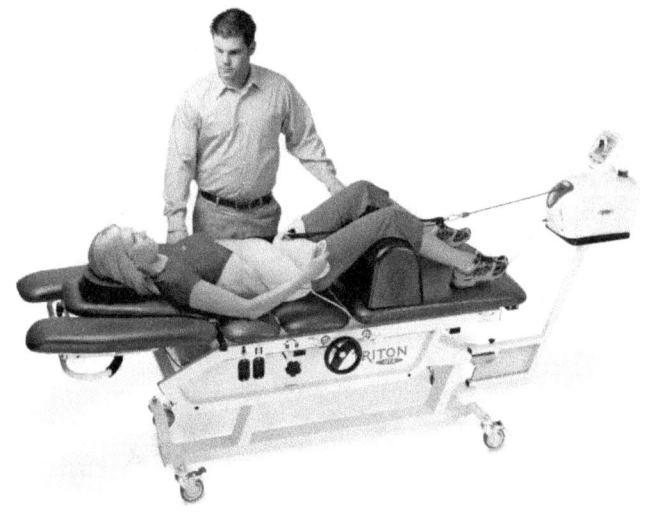

For cervical (neck) SDT smaller forces are used, but the patient is positioned in the unit's cervical device which gently pulls using cranial bolsters.

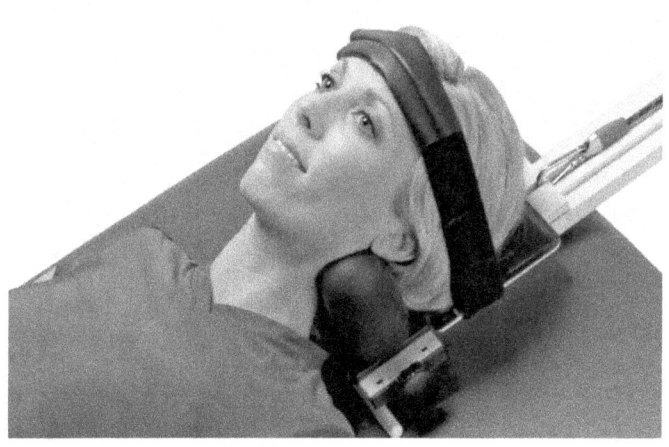

Here's what our SDT table looks like when used for cervical SDT. Don't worry, it's very gentle. Just look at her smiling.

The bottom line is that SDT, when applied appropriately, can not only feel awesome, but it can encourage some real healing. My patients love it and I bet you would too!

Chapter 13

Getting Back to the Basics of Wellness

Case Study

Molly was one of the worse neuropathy cases that I took on. She told us that she could not feel her feet at all and that her medications "make me sleepy, tired and gain weight." She described her foot symptoms as burning, tingling, numbness, and cold feeling. "The underside of my feet feels sore but, at the same time, I don't feel them. It feels like my feet are encapsulated in ice – like Frankenstein feet. They keep me up at night while trying to sleep. It was preventing me from walking around my house doing anything because my feet hurt so badly, and they were either ice cold or burning up and I felt like there were thousands of needles in them, poking me. I couldn't walk without terrible pain."

At first, I told her that I could NOT accept her into the program because our testing indicated that she had over 90% loss of the sensory nerves in her feet. She had a very arthritic spine, was obese, lethargic, on 9 different prescription medications and had multiple other medical diagnoses. I told her and her husband that I thought it was too late in her case. They persisted, and I finally accepted her, but said she'd have to do the whole program 100%. She said she would and she really did.

Here's what Molly had to say on her final evaluation. "I notice a great difference in the feeling in my feet now than I did before, because I can actually feel them. I don't have the pins and needles that I had. It's much better walking. I take bigger steps and I'm more confident when I walk and now I'm beginning to feel like myself, like 15 years ago."

"I didn't know it, but I was walking curved over and now my shoulders are down, and they feel much better and I just feel better all over. I have a better posture. My husband said that he sees me [walking better]. I'd been taking one step at a time since 1988. I couldn't even do housework because of the combination of my shoulder and the feet; I was just in a terrible position. I was mentally depressed."

"I would recommend anyone who thinks they have a nerve problem like neuropathy to come to (Dr. Prax) because even my attitude has improved. I've lost close to 30 pounds and I'm going to continue losing weight. I think if your whole body works together you feel better and your program brings it all together."

Molly R.

For a moment, think back to when you were a kid. Chances are that back in elementary school, you had boundless energy. The days were long but it didn't matter you could probably run around the neighborhood with your friends with hardly a thought of food, pain, or fatigue.

Now, maybe you have kids or grandkids, and you watch them go at playtime for hours without a pause – and it's exhausting! We joke about bottling all that energy. We get nostalgic about feeling limitless and free, but not enough of us know that there really is a way to regain some of those powerful feelings again.

Wellness is very personal and means different things to different people in terms of preferences and outcomes:

- If you have debilitating back pain, you might feel powerful again if you could get through the day without taking prescription painkillers and suffering through their side effects.
- If your arthritis restricts your daily physical activities, you might feel powerful again if you could go for a hike, or knit another afghan without it resulting in days of excruciating joint pain.
- If you suffer from peripheral neuropathy, you might feel powerful again if you could regain

sensation in your fingertips and take up the activities and hobbies you left behind years ago.

Getting older isn't for the meek – but remember that we are lucky to have made it this far!

So, what will it take for you to feel energetic and powerful again? There is no blanket answer to that question. Every person presents with their own set of symptoms, conditions, and preferences. Each person has their own set of goals that will make them feel healthy and happy. All of that makes it complicated to prescribe a roadmap to wellness.

As we discussed in prior chapters, we offer several healing modalities in our office that patients with chronic pain find to be beneficial. Brain-Based Therapy, vibration, low-light laser therapy, and electrotherapy are a few important resources that many of our patients use every day. We also counsel our patients about the importance of eating a well-balanced diet.

Good nutrition should be considered the cornerstone of any wellness plan. The food you use to fuel your body will make a huge difference when your cells need to repair and regenerate themselves. We promote a diet that's big on unprocessed foods, fruits, vegetables, and natural protein sources. Eating like this gives your body the vitamins, minerals, and antioxidants it needs to stay strong and healthy.

What Else Can I Do to Feel Well?

Exercise: A Conundrum Wrapped Around an Enigma

I often hear patients lament about the fact that they cannot workout due to the pain in their feet. This is what I would call a conundrum wrapped around an enigma. We know from experience and research that exercise helps stimulate so many things, including the immune system, circulation, muscle growth, nerves, and brain. Exercise actually has been shown to decrease pain but how are you supposed to exercise when it feels like you're walking on gravel or pushpins? It's nearly impossible but, somehow, we must find a way to push through.

What I usually encourage is for a patient to start with a super clean, anti-inflammatory diet combined with the recommended at-home therapies and then, when feeling good enough, begin some form of exercise. Start with exercises that are very light such as cycling, swimming, water aerobics, gentle yoga, (even chair yoga), stretching classes or tai chi. The challenge is starting. We are going to feel pain whether we exercise or not so we might as well do something positive.

YouTube is an excellent source. If you Google "chair yoga", you'll get over 26 million results! Hint: you only need one or two, so don't be overwhelmed. Just start. Give something a try. Start with only one posture and see how it feels. Progress from there. My personal favorite Yoga Channel is "Yoga with Adriene" (https://www.youtube.com/user/yogawithadriene). Again, swimming, or anything in the water, is very gentle and you can get a heck of a workout too!

I'll be honest, as a triathlete, I workout all the time and, most of the time, I love it. But there are times (often at 5:30 in the morning) when I'd rather do something else (like sleep), and every time I push myself to go to the gym or to get on the road, I thank myself later because I feel so good after the workout. I feel good because I did my workout, and my body feels better too. There is also a sense of pride that "I did it!" I promise, you'll feel the same things too – start now!

Chiropractic Care

At the heart of our practice is a busy wellness clinic that offers chiropractic care, nutrition, and education. We strongly believe in the power of a strong, aligned spine that supports a healthy nervous system. Keeping the spine aligned is achieved through gentle, routine adjustments. For most of our patients, one adjustment a month works great. But patients recovering from an accident, illness, infection, or injury sometimes require more frequent adjustments for a period of time.

Regular chiropractic adjustments cannot only improve the health of your spine and nervous system, but they can also:

- improve mood
- improve sleep

- increase energy
- decrease pain
- boost flexibility
- stop recurring headaches

One of the most important things adjustments do is boost the immune system. This is accomplished by clearing the neural pathways so that the central nervous system can communicate effectively with the immune system (and every other system in your body). This communication is hindered when the spine experiences subluxations, which are misalignments along the spinal column. When the nervous system's pathways are cleared, the effects can be quite powerful:

- decrease in colds, flu, and other contagious illnesses
- greatly reduce the symptoms of asthma and allergies
- result in fewer hospital admissions

Unfortunately, most people only think to go to the chiropractor if their back hurts. But we can do so much more than just fix back pain!

What Do Chiropractic Adjustments Have To Do with Peripheral Neuropathy?

As you may recall, the treatment modalities we already discussed for peripheral neuropathy were all about rebuilding nerves, growing blood vessels, and improving muscle function. Well, chiropractic adjustments are all about clearing the way for the nervous system to do its job correctly. So, when your brain can tell those tiny nerve endings that it's time to regrow, all those other efforts we talked about are far more likely to be successful.

In addition to fostering the regrowth of damaged nerves, adjustments can also "un-pinch" nerves. A pinched nerve can cause numbness and pain, just like peripheral neuropathy. Getting the bones back into their proper places takes pressure off of nerves, alleviates pain, and promotes a healthy, active lifestyle. It also gets the joint in the hands, feet or both, moving better if they are affected by neuropathy.

What Should I Do if I Suspect That I Have Peripheral Neuropathy?

The National Institutes of Neurological Disorders and Stroke says that peripheral neuropathy affects roughly 24 million Americans.[27] It's a very common condition among people in certain populations, such as diabetics, cancer patients, and those taking statin medications to lower their cholesterol. Therefore, it's important to

---

[27] Ferreira, Leonor Mateus. "Chiropractic Care May Help Control Peripheral Neuropathy in Diabetics." Diabetes News Journal. N.p., 16 Mar. 2015. Web. 27 July 2015. <http://diabetesnewsjournal.com/2015/03/17/chiropractic-care-may-help-control-peripheral-neuropathy-in-diabetics/>.

know that if you do have peripheral neuropathy, you are certainly not alone.

While the early stages of the symptoms may seem to be just minor irritations, early diagnosis of peripheral neuropathy can prevent the condition from becoming worse. Talk to your doctor or chiropractor right away to diagnose and determine the cause of your peripheral neuropathy. There could be ways to change your medical treatment plan that can reduce your symptoms.

We also strongly recommend visiting our office as soon as you can. We may be able to offer you a variety of treatments that can reduce or even eliminate the pain, numbness, and tingling associated with peripheral neuropathy. There is no reason to wait until the problem becomes worse – as soon as you suspect that something is wrong, seek professional help. It's the best way to ensure your health and wellness for many years to come.

Don't Be "THAT" Guy

I fell in love with the sport of triathlon in early 2014. At first, it was just a great chance to work out with my two sons, Blaze and Jordan, but that quickly turned into a passion for the sport of swimming, biking, and running. Looking back, I knew so little about running, and even less about swimming. My biking experience consisted of periodic trail riding with the boys. It's amazing that I was able to *complete* my first sprint triathlon in 2014.

Fast forward one and half years to mid-season 2015. My mind was that of a 14 or even 16-year-old (like my boys) yet my body was that of a man in his mid-40s. To think that I could actually compete, or even keep up with these guys! I remember telling friends and patients that "they are getting so fast, I feel like I have to work out twice as hard to even be half as fast". So that's exactly what I did. I cranked up the training.

Not only was I training 6-7 days per week (sometimes two in a day), I reasoned that I needed to get my running speed up as it was my slowest sport. The boys were getting faster and faster. At this point, I couldn't keep up with Jordan, the 16-year-old. On the other hand, Blaze, the 14-year-old and I, were quite competitive. In a race in 2015, I beat him by just 3 seconds! A race that took over an hour and I beat him by 3 little seconds!

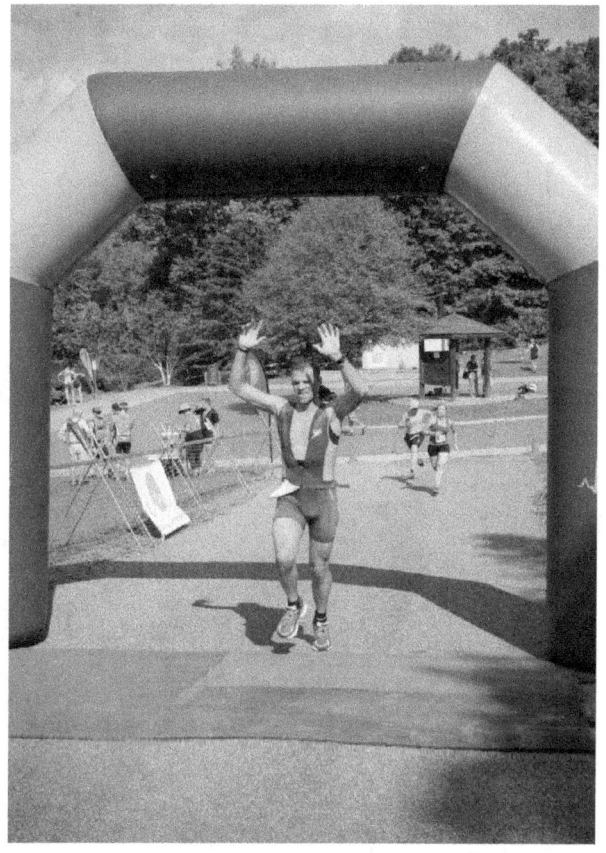

I felt like I nearly suffered a heart attack too! Look at my face. See the kid with the hat and head tucked?

I remember it was after that race that I began feeling this weird right thigh pain. It typically came on after 5 miles of running or really hard biking. It even started hurting after sitting in a chair, especially on our kitchen stools.

Well, being a doctor, I self-diagnosed a muscle strain and treated it as such. I tried massage, more massage, then deep tissue massage, and even Rolfing (a system of deep manipulation of soft/connective tissue). I tried stretching, yoga, and even taking a week off here and there. I tried applying arnica and other creams, Epsom salt baths and anything else I could think of for this "muscle pain" that just wouldn't go away.

It was getting so chronic and was just not going away, so I finally decided that I should go see an expert, a doctor who specializes in running and sports injuries. At this point my training was hampered; I had missed a few races and had cut out running completely.

So, I was motivated – I scheduled an appointment. Well, exactly 73 hours before the appointment (72 hours is the required time before canceling an appointment without a charge) I called and canceled it. I reasoned, "What does this doctor know that I don't know? I already know what it is – it's a muscle spasm or muscle strain. It just needs more time or massage – it probably needs more stretching."

Well two months later, in November, I'm still suffering from the same symptoms and it's not getting any better. Having missed half of the 2015 season, and now I have the 2016 season coming up, I decided I should reschedule and go see this doctor. Well, what do you think would happen 73 hours before that second appointment? That's right, yours truly, "Mr. Know it all," decided to cancel the appointment. I used the same logic as I did the last time. "What does he know?"

Fortunately, my wife – aka "my better half" – gently suggested, "Why don't you just go see what he has to say?" So, I kept the appointment and reluctantly went down to the University of Virginia to see Dr. Robert Wilder, the running expert.

He swiftly and confidently performed a detailed examination of my leg, my posture, and my gait. He did tests that I've never seen before. Then, he sent me down to get an x-ray of my leg. Within 20 minutes the results were back, he popped it up on the screen and from across the room it was glaring at me – I had a stress fracture in my femur.

Who fractures the femur – the strongest bone in the body!? Well, apparently, I do and my recovery time would be a full six weeks off of running and then a very slow return-to-running regimen. Guess what? That solved my problem and even though I missed a few races in 2016, I was back on my feet again.

Why do I tell this story? It's to make a point and here it is: don't be "THAT GUY!"

That guy who thinks he or she knows what their problem is and how to fix it. I was "that guy" and obviously, I was not the expert on running injuries. I wasted almost 6 months of my training and triathlon career getting slower and slower because I didn't reach out to an expert, the person who knows about injuries like mine.

Don't be "that guy" with your neuropathy either. If you've worked with your doctor for more than six months and still haven't gotten any results, s/he's not gonna figure it out; trust me. That would be like going to a psychiatrist to figure out a broken bone...wrong practitioner! Get yourself to an expert. Find a doctor who specializes in peripheral neuropathy. Somebody who has a proven track record with this tricky condition.

You need to get working on this now because every day of the wrong treatment (or even no treatment) gets you closer and closer to permanent nerve damage. At some point, if it keeps progressing, it will be irreversible and no one will be able to help you – not even my program.

Get this taken care of before it sucks more and more joy out of your life. This is no way to live. Reach out to me and my team. I'd love to see if we can help you out. If you (or someone you know) is out of our area, not to worry, s/he may qualify for my remote program where we can use technology like Skype, Facebook, email and the telephone to get the help that is needed. Now is the time to start your recovery (or even see if recovery is possible). Here's my office number 434-977-5433 and my email is info@chroniccarecharlottesville.com.

I'll See You on YouTube

I have a YouTube channel that covers a lot of the material in this book and it is constantly being added to and upgraded. As of the printing of this book I have over 350 videos, most of which are specifically on Reversing Peripheral Neuropathy. As I find a new study, or have an inspirational story to share, or find a new piece of technology, I cut a video on it. In this "Information Age," it's all about sharing and that's what I do.

Make sure to go to my YouTube channel to keep abreast of Reversing Neuropathy. It's simple to do. Just go to YouTube.com and type in "Dr. Brian Prax" and you'll be led right to my channel. Hit the subscribe button (it's the little red button at the bottom of the video and IT'S FREE!) and start watching. Hey, if you like my video, hit the "like" button or write me a comment or question; I'll reply...I really will!

Chapter 14

Testimonials

J udith sought treatment in our office for occasional sharp discomfort in her pubic and abdominal regions that would increase with movement and improve with rest. She had been through every possible diagnostic test to determine what was causing this intense, relentless pain. Ultrasound, X-ray, MRI, CAT scans, some of them multiple times. Every single time the test would come back normal. At the time she came in to see me her doctor was pushing her to do an "exploratory surgery." He was out of testing procedures and figured he'd need to open her up and take a look in there.

She rated her discomfort at a 7 on a pain scale of 1-10 with 10 being the highest. Her tummy pain was so bad just standing and walking was a very painful chore. Shopping was a nightmare for her. A little history digging also revealed that she had eczema and balance problems.

I put on my dietary program and used a variety of hands on therapies to help her balance and abdominal pain. She started her program in the late summer and every time she came to office she was complaining about abdominal pain. Little by little the complaints lessened and by October, the trend of complaints came to a complete stop.

In November we asked her how she was doing and she told me that she had no pain in her abdomen for nearly 2 months. She also said, "I lost 11 pounds...the pain in my abdomen is gone after doing the detox and following Dr. Brian's dietary recommendations. My eczema is completely gone and my balance has improved. I have reaped a lot of rewards from the program."

You know what it was? A gluten sensitivity. The solution wasn't more testing or more drugs, and it certainly wasn't an exploratory surgery, it was to stop the offending food that her body was reacting to.

"I went hiking at humpback rock. No walking sticks. Feeling the earth beneath my feet again. My balance is much improved. They have miracle workers at Dr. Prax's. Much hard work and dedication got me the results I needed for my peripheral neuropathy."

Linda M.

"My fingers were numb and my legs were having sciatica. They were keeping me up all night. It was just pain and aching. The diet is more like a lifestyle. It's watching what I put in my mouth. I'm eating real human food. I have lost 7 pounds in about four weeks. I am more alert, I am not having my gastrointestinal problems. At six weeks into a 12-week program, I am feeling 50% better. I'm very pleased with my progress. It turns out that

we can regenerate nerves – most people don't do that. Their physicians don't tell them what's possible because they don't even know themselves."

Mary P

"I was on metformin and gabapentin for a year; they didn't seem to do anything. Thanks to your program it has made a big difference. I started out with diabetes and then reversed it with your diet and supplements. I am learning to eat the right foods instead of everything the government tells us is great for us. It wasn't easy. The symptoms started with tingling and then lead to numbness – no feeling at all. Now I have come to the point, using the Rebuilder and the diet, I am getting some nerve endings renewed. I have a better sense of feeling in my hands and feet. I can walk better, I can walk further. I've lost 40 pounds and it has given me a new lease on life."

Bill M.

"I tried medications including Neurontin. My doctor told me there was nothing they could really do. At Chronic Care Charlottesville, I learned how to eat better and take care of myself. I can say that I am 100% better. I feel better all over."

Francis D

"I absolutely love the detox. It makes you feel wonderful. It's not a cookie-cutter program. It's customized to the person and what works best for them. I love the orthotics, I love the cervical pillow. Dr. Brian gave wonderful facts and advice. I was having a lot of pain; so bad that I couldn't even get off the floor, but since I've come to see Dr. Brian I am so much better."

Peg L

"I couldn't sleep at all and my anxiety was high. I couldn't relax and it was a constant worry. I'm psyched! I don't have to worry anymore. The pain is gone. I feel like $1 million most days. There's always something to be happy about. I feel relieved. I can now see myself back in a routine of exercise. My balance is much better. I don't have to worry so much about falling over. Give it a shot. You've got to try it. You'll get support and an increased knowledge base of what you can do for yourself. I really enjoyed this process".

Celina P

"After 31 visits, I was 90-95% cured."

–Bill G

"After only 2 treatments I was able to sleep at night without socks which had been one of my big problems, because my feet had been so cold."

–Mickey W.

"I was taking pain medication every day, after 12 visits I stopped taking pain medication. I had no symptoms at night and I did not need sleeping aids anymore. I am extremely happy with my choice to begin the program."

–Rosanna V.

"I have gone from 44% sensory loss down to 15% sensory loss halfway through the program. I'm getting better and I feel a whole lot better."

–Kim M.

"I saw an ad for neuropathy which intrigued me because I was developing neuropathy in my feet and legs. I saw my podiatrist and he confirmed that I have neuropathy. So, I decided to try the program; I had always had trouble with my legs particularly. I could not sleep at night because my legs bothered me so much – in less than 2 weeks I was beginning to sleep through the night!"

–Bob B.

"I came here because of the numbness in my feet; it was all over the top and bottom of my feet, as well as my toes. I've been on the program awhile now and all I have is a little bit of numbness, so it is definitely working. I would encourage anyone to come here and visit with them. I have been very happy and I believe their maintenance program will help me as well!"

–Matt B.

"Over 5 years ago, I was told by a well-respected neurologist that "nothing can be done other than to take B12 and be careful not to fall". I heard about this program at a local Rotary meeting, thought I would give it a try...fully expecting a similar situation because of my age. To my surprise, after testing, I knew there was potential that I could really get some help. I am now in my 8th week of therapy and the results have been amazing. I no longer have the tingling sensation or pain."

–Burnell S.

"I have been coming here for about a week and a half now. Since then I have lost nine pounds sticking to the nutrition plan. I have such bad feet problems, back pain, neck pain, and hand pain. That's why I decided to come. Since I've been coming, I have already seen quite a bit of difference in this short amount of time. I can't believe the progress I've had in such a short amount of time."

–Ann R.

"My feet have been dead for quite some time. Two different times in my pick-up, I couldn't feel my accelerator. We started the treatment and about 3-4 weeks into the program, after beginning the home treatment...I could feel the carpet when I was walking and that was the first time I had done that in quite some time."

–Mark O.

"I was having pretty bad neuropathy and it was continuing to get worse after seeing medical doctors. They were just giving me some pain pills and vitamin B12 shots. I decided I needed to do something better & be proactive. This will be my third week and between all the treatments they do here, I am already improving – I'm down to one incident a week and I was having 5-6 incidents a day."

–Kelly C.

"Neuropathy was affecting my life pretty bad for almost a year, to the point where I was in pain most of the time. Since I've been coming here for 3 or 4 sessions now, I have already noticed a lot of difference and I am already feeling a lot better.

–Jesse R.

"I came here very apprehensive. I have been coming only a few weeks now and I have already regained so much strength in my left leg, which was the problem. I barely use my cane at all now – just for a little security. I just can't believe how well I am doing after only being treated for a short amount of time!"

–Dorothy C.

"I have suffered from neuropathy for at least three years. I have been completing treatment here and it has already been successful. I can sleep at night without my feet burning and hurting!"

–Betty P.

Reversing Neuropathy

"I have been coming about five weeks and I can already tell some improvement in the bottom of my feet."

–Gary C.

"I am relatively new to the program; this is only my third visit. I have already gone from a pain level of 8 to a pain level of 2!"

– Kim N.

"I have been coming about 6 weeks. When I came in, I had severe pain all the way from my hip down to my big toe. As of today, I am able to wiggle my big toe and I have feeling in it! I have NO more pain in my hips or legs. Overall, my time spent here has been well worthwhile! I must say that the staff has been very professional, helpful, and encouraging."

–Nell M.

"I am in the third week of my treatment, when I came in, my left foot was killing me and my right foot was not far behind it. I was asked to rate my pain on a level of 1 – 10 during my consultation, and I have been at a level 10 for about three or four months now. My pain level now is nearly gone completely."

–James F.

"I came here after seeing the ad in the paper. I decided to come in because of my neuropathy being so bad. It took a little bit of work but everything they have done here for me has been very great. The staff here is very nice, which helps a lot when coming in for treatment."

–Everisto M.

www.ingramcontent.com/pod-product-compliance
Lightning Source LLC
Chambersburg PA
CBHW071306220526
45468CB00001B/286